T0294576

PAIN MEDICINE
A CASE-BASED LEARNING SERIES

The Wrist and Hand

PAIN MEDICINE
A CASE-BASED LEARNING SERIES

The Wrist and Hand

STEVEN D. WALDMAN, MD, JD

ELSEVIER

Elsevier
1600 John F. Kennedy Blvd.
Ste 1800
Philadelphia, PA 19103-2899

PAIN MEDICINE: A CASE-BASED LEARNING SERIES   ISBN: 978-0-323-83453-7
THE WRIST AND HAND

Notice

Practitioners and researchers must always rely on their own experience and knowledge in evaluating and using any information, methods, compounds or experiments described herein. Because of rapid advances in the medical sciences, in particular, independent verification of diagnoses and drug dosages should be made. To the fullest extent of the law, no responsibility is assumed by Elsevier, authors, editors or contributors for any injury and/or damage to persons or property as a matter of products liability, negligence or otherwise, or from any use or operation of any methods, products, instructions, or ideas contained in the material herein.

Executive Content Strategist: Michael Houston
Content Development Specialist: Jeannine Carrado/Laura Klein
Director, Content Development: Ellen Wurm-Cutter
Publishing Services Manager: Shereen Jameel
Senior Project Manager: Karthikeyan Murthy
Design Direction: Amy Buxton

Printed in India.

Last digit is the print number: 9 8 7 6 5 4 3 2 1

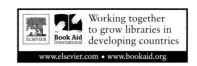

Working together to grow libraries in developing countries

www.elsevier.com • www.bookaid.org

"When you go after honey with a balloon, the great thing is to not let the bees know you're coming."

WINNIE THE POOH

It's Harder Than It Looks
MAKING THE CASE FOR CASE-BASED LEARNING

For the sake of full disclosure, I was one of those guys. You know, the ones who wax poetic about how hard it is to teach our students how to do procedures. Let me tell you, teaching folks how to do epidurals on women in labor certainly takes its toll on the coronary arteries. It's true, I am amazing . . . I am great . . . I have nerves of steel. Yes, I could go on like this for hours . . . but you have heard it all before. But, it's again that time of year when our new students sit eagerly before us, full of hope and dreams . . . and that harsh reality comes slamming home . . . it is a lot harder to teach beginning medical students "doctoring" than it looks.

A few years ago, I was asked to teach first-year medical and physician assistant students how to take a history and perform a basic physical exam. In my mind this should be easy, no big deal, I won't have to do much more than show up. After all, I was the guy who wrote that amazing book on physical diagnosis. After all, I had been teaching medical students, residents, and fellows how to do highly technical (and dangerous, I might add) interventional pain management procedures since seemingly right after the Civil War. Seriously, it was no big deal . . . I could do it in my sleep . . . with one arm tied behind my back . . . blah . . . blah . . . blah.

For those of you who have had the privilege of teaching "doctoring," you already know what I am going to say next. *It's harder than it looks!* Let me repeat this to disabuse any of you who, like me, didn't get it the first time. *It is harder than it looks!* I only had to meet with my first-year medical and physician assistant students a couple of times to get it through my thick skull: **It really is harder than it looks**. In case you are wondering, the reason that our students look back at us with those blank, confused, bored, and ultimately dismissive looks is simple: They lack context. That's right, they lack the context to understand what we are talking about.

It's really that simple . . . or hard . . . depending on your point of view or stubbornness, as the case may be. To understand why context is king, you have to look only as far as something as basic as the Review of Systems. The Review of Systems is about as basic as it gets, yet why is it so perplexing to our students? Context. I guess it should come as no surprise to anyone that the student is completely lost when you talk about . . . let's say . . . the "constitutional" portion of the Review of Systems, without the context of what a specific constitutional finding, say a fever or chills, might mean to a patient. If you tell the student that you need to ask about fever, chills, and the other "constitutional" stuff and you take it no further, you might as well be talking about the International Space

Station. Just save your breath; it makes absolutely no sense to your students. Yes, they want to please, so they will memorize the elements of the Review of Systems, but that is about as far as it goes. On the other hand, if you present the case of Jannette Patton, a 28-year-old first-year medical resident with a fever and headache, you can see the lights start to come on. By the way, this is what Jannette looks like, and as you can see, Jannette is sicker than a dog. This, at its most basic level, is what *Case-Based Learning* is all about.

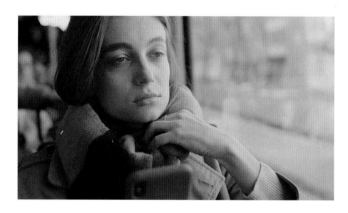

I would like to tell you that, smart guy that I am, I immediately saw the light and became a convert to *Case-Based Learning*. But truth be told, it was COVID-19 that really got me thinking about *Case-Based Learning*. Before the COVID-19 pandemic, I could just drag the students down to the med/surg wards and walk into a patient room and riff. Everyone was a winner. For the most part, the patients loved to play along and thought it was cool. The patient and the bedside was all I needed to provide the context that was necessary to illustrate what I was trying to teach—the "why headache and fever don't mix" kind of stuff. Had COVID-19 not rudely disrupted my ability to teach at the bedside, I suspect that you would not be reading this *Preface*, as I would not have had to write it. Within a very few days after the COVID-19 pandemic hit, my days of bedside teaching disappeared, but my students still needed context. This got me focused on how to provide the context they needed. The answer was, of course, *Case-Based Learning*. What started as a desire to provide context . . . because it really was **harder than it looked** . . . led me to begin work on this eight-volume *Case-Based Learning* textbook series. What you will find within these volumes are a bunch of fun, real-life cases that help make each patient come alive for the student. These cases provide the contextual teaching points that make it easy for the teacher to explain why, when Jannette's chief complaint is *"My head is killing me and I've got a fever,"* it is a big deal.

Have fun!

Steven D. Waldman, MD, JD
Spring 2021

ACKNOWLEDGMENTS

A very special thanks to my editors, Michael Houston PhD, Jeannine Carrado, and Karthikeyan Murthy, for all of their hard work and perseverance in the face of disaster. Great editors such as Michael, Jeannine, and Karthikeyan make their authors look great, for they not only understand how to bring the Three Cs of great writing...Clarity + Consistency + Conciseness...to the author's work, but unlike me, they can actually punctuate and spell!

Steven D. Waldman, MD, JD

P.S....Sorry for all the ellipses, guys!

CONTENTS

Harry Boyden

A 58-Year-Old Male With Right Wrist Pain

- Learn the common causes of wrist pain.
- Develop an understanding of the unique anatomy of the wrist joint.
- Develop an understanding of the causes of arthritis of the wrist joint.
- Learn the clinical presentation of osteoarthritis of the wrist joint.
- Learn how to use physical examination to identify pathology associated with wrist pain.
- Develop an understanding of the treatment options for osteoarthritis of the wrist joint.
- Learn the appropriate testing options to help diagnose osteoarthritis of the wrist joint.
- Learn to identify red flags in patients who present with wrist pain.
- Develop an understanding of the role in interventional pain management in the treatment of wrist pain.

Harry Boyden

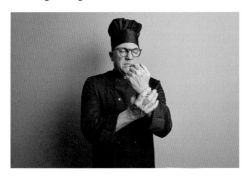

Harry Boyden is a 58-year-old chef with the chief complaint of "my right wrist is killing me." Harry went on to say that he wouldn't have bothered coming in, but he was getting where he couldn't hold a fry pan in his right hand because his wrist hurt so much. I asked Harry if he had anything like this happen before. He shook his head and responded, "Just my feet. You can't stand on that hard kitchen floor all day long and not have your feet hurt by the end of the day. Doctor, I can live with the feet—sore feet are just an occupational hazard. Usually I just take a couple of Motrin and give them a good soak, and that will usually set me right after a day or so. What worries me this time is that this damn right wrist is hurting all the time, especially when I try to pick up a fry pan and toss the food so it won't burn, something I used to do about 1000 times a day. Now just the weight of the pan when I lift it really hurts, but that flick of the wrist that you need to toss the food and then catch it hurts so bad that I have been working the pass so I don't drop a hot pan and burn myself or someone around me. This is a real problem. I'm pretty tough, but this really has me worried because at my age executive chef jobs aren't that easy to come by. I worked my whole life to get where I am, and I don't want this stupid wrist pain to cut my career short! I don't want to go back to being a line cook. Like everybody else in the food industry, if I don't work, I don't eat. The other thing is, this damn wrist has my sleep all jacked up. Even when I am sleeping, every time I move my wrist the damn pain wakes me up! Hell, some mornings, I have to brush my teeth with my left hand."

I asked Harry about any antecedent trauma and he just shook his head. "Doc, this kind of snuck up on me. At first, my wrist had this deep ache that would get better with some Motrin and rest. Over the last 6 weeks, the Motrin just quit working. But Doc, like I said, I gotta work." I asked Harry what made his pain worse and he said, "Any time he used his wrist, it hurt like hell."

I asked Harry to point with one finger to show me where it hurts the most. He grabbed his right wrist and said, "Doc, I can't really point to one place. It kind of hurts all over. And you know, the crazy thing is, sometimes I feel like the wrist is popping." I asked if he had any fever or chills and he shook his head no. "What about steroids?" I asked. "Did you ever take any cortisone or drugs like that?" Harry again shook his head no and replied, "Too many drunks and stoners in the food industry as it is." I laughed, then said that maybe it was a time to stop eating out. Harry smiled and said, "Doc, you're safe when I'm the one cooking for you and yours. Get my wrist better and I will cook you a meal to remember!"

On physical examination, Harry was afebrile. His respirations were 18 and his pulse was 74 and regular. His blood pressure (BP) was slightly elevated at 142/84. I made a note to recheck it again before he left the office. His head, eyes, ears, nose, throat (HEENT) exam was normal, as was his cardiopulmonary examination. His thyroid was normal. His abdominal examination revealed no abnormal mass or organomegaly. There was no costovertebral angle (CVA) tenderness. There was no peripheral edema. His low back examination was unremarkable. I did a rectal exam, which revealed no mass and a normal prostate. Visual inspection of the right wrist revealed no cutaneous lesions or obvious mass. The wrist was slightly warm to touch, but there was no obvious infection or swelling. Palpation of the right wrist revealed mild diffuse tenderness, with no obvious effusion or point tenderness (Fig. 1.1). There was mild crepitus, but I did not appreciate any popping. Range of motion was decreased with pain exacerbated with flexion and extension of the wrist. The tuck sign for extensor tenosynovitis was negative bilaterally (Fig. 1.2). The left wrist examination was normal, as was examination of his other major joints, other than some mild osteoarthritis in the right hand. A careful neurologic examination of the upper extremities revealed no evidence of peripheral or entrapment neuropathy, and the deep tendon reflexes were normal.

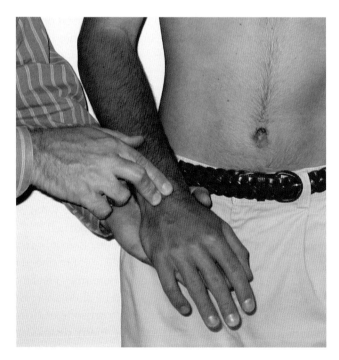

Fig. 1.1 Palpation of the dorsal aspect of the wrist. (From Waldman S. *Physical Diagnosis of Pain: An Atlas of Signs and Symptoms*. 4th ed. Philadelphia: Elsevier; 2021 [Fig. 108-1].)

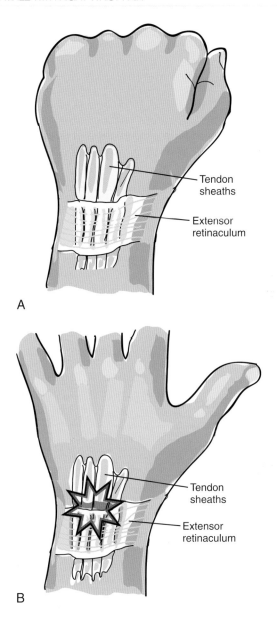

Fig. 1.2 The Tuck sign for extensor tenosynovitis of the wrist. (A) To elicit a Tuck sign, the examiner has the patient lightly clench the fist for 30 seconds. The examiner observes the dorsum of the clenched fist for swelling that is consistent with extensor tenosynovitis. (B) The examiner has the patient gradually fully extend the fingers of the clenched fist. The Tuck sign for extensor tenosynovitis of the wrist is considered positive if the patient extends the hand, and the area of swelling moves proximally then folds under the flexor retinaculum like a sheet being tucked under a mattress. (From Waldman S. *Physical Diagnosis of Pain: An Atlas of Signs and Symptoms*. 3rd ed. St. Louis: Elsevier; 2016 [Figs. 118-1, 118-2].)

Key Clinical Points—What's Important and What's Not

THE HISTORY

- No history of acute trauma
- No history of previous significant wrist pain
- No fever or chills
- Gradual onset of wrist pain with exacerbation of pain with wrist use
- Popping sensation in the right wrist
- Sleep disturbance
- Difficulty using the wrist both at work and to provide self-care

THE PHYSICAL EXAMINATION

- Patient is afebrile
- Normal visual inspection of wrist
- Palpation of right wrist reveals diffuse tenderness
- No point tenderness
- No increased temperature of right wrist
- Crepitus to palpation (see Fig. 1.1)
- Tuck test for extensor tenosynovitis was negative (see Fig. 1.2)

OTHER FINDINGS OF NOTE

- Slightly elevated BP
- Normal HEENT examination
- Normal cardiovascular examination
- Normal pulmonary examination
- Normal abdominal examination
- No peripheral edema
- Normal upper extremity neurologic examination, motor and sensory examination
- Examination of other joints normal

 ## What Tests Would You Like to Order?

The following tests were ordered:
- Plain radiographs of the right wrist

TEST RESULTS

The plain radiographs of the right wrist revealed severe pancarpal osteoarthritis (Fig. 1.3).

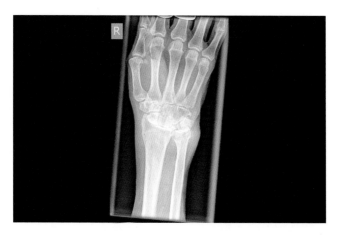

Fig. 1.3 Arthritis of the carpal joints. (From Islam SU, Brown D, Cheung G. Management of osteoarthritis of the wrist and hand. *Orthopaed Trauma*. 2019;33(1):30–37 [Fig. 4]. ISSN 1877-1327, https://doi.org/10.1016/j.mporth.2018.11.012, http://www.sciencedirect.com/science/article/pii/S1877132718301672.)

Clinical Correlation—Putting It All Together

What is the diagnosis?
- Osteoarthritis of the right wrist

The Science Behind the Diagnosis

ANATOMY OF THE JOINTS OF THE WRIST

In humans, the wrist functions to transfer the forces and motions of the hand to the forearm and proximal upper extremity. The wrist allows movement in three planes:
1. Flexion/extension
2. Radial/ulnar deviation
3. Pronation/supination
   To understand the functional anatomy of the wrist, it is important for the clinician to understand that the wrist is not a single joint but in fact is a complex of five separate joints or compartments that work in concert to allow humans to carry out their activities of daily living (Figs. 1.4 and 1.5). These five joints are:
1. The distal radioulnar joint, which is composed of the distal radius and ulna and their interosseous membrane
2. The radiocarpal joint, which is composed of the distal radius and the proximal surfaces of the scaphoid and lunate bones
3. The ulnar carpal joint, which is composed of the distal ulna and the triangular fibroelastic cartilage whose function is to connect the distal ulna with the lunate and triquetrum

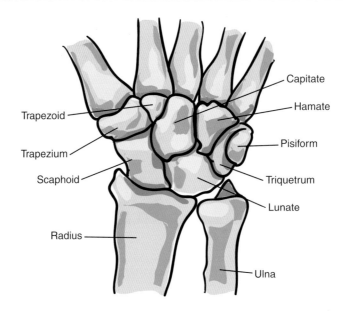

Fig. 1.4 Bony anatomy of the wrist. (From Waldman S. *Physical Diagnosis of Pain: An Atlas of Signs and Symptoms*. 4th ed. Philadelphia: Elsevier; 2021 [Fig. 106-1].)

4. The proximal carpal joints, which connect the scaphoid, lunate, and triquetrum via the dorsal, palmar, and interosseous ligaments
5. The midcarpal joints, which are composed of the capitate, hamate, trapezium, and trapezoid bones

The interaction of the many osseous elements that make up the wrist is made possible by a complex collection of ligamentous structures and a unique structure called the triangular fibroelastic cartilage (TFC) (see Fig. 1.5). In general, the ligaments can be thought of as being intrinsic to the wrist (i.e., having their origin and insertion on the carpal bones) or extrinsic to the wrist (i.e., having their origin on the distal radius or ulna and insertion on the carpal bones). All of the ligaments of the wrist have in common a close proximity to the bones of the wrist, which increases their ability to transfer force to the forearm and proximal upper extremity. This lack of interposing muscle and/or soft tissue also makes the ligamentous structures of the wrist—the nerves, blood vessels, and bones beneath them—more susceptible to injury.

THE CLINICAL SYNDROME

Arthritis of the wrist is a common complaint that can cause significant pain and suffering. The wrist joint is susceptible to the development of arthritis from various conditions that have in common the ability to damage joint cartilage.

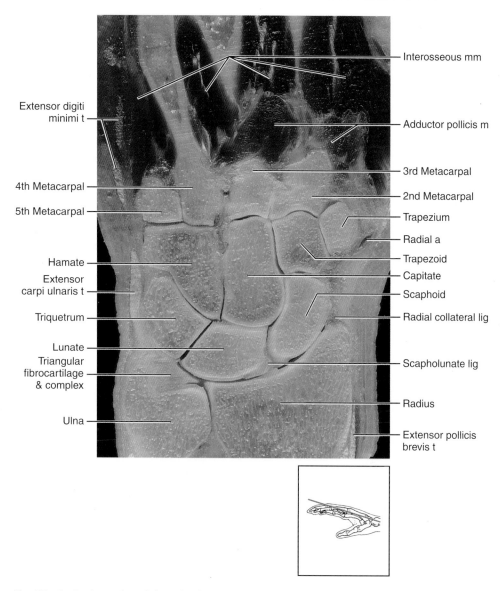

Fig. 1.5 Anatomic section of the wrist demonstrating joints and the triangular fibroelastic cartilage. (From Kang HS, Ahn JM, Resnick D. *MRI of the Extremities*. 2nd ed. Philadelphia: Saunders; 2002:163.)

Patients with arthritis of the wrist present with pain, swelling, and decreasing function of the wrist. Decreased grip strength is also a common finding. Osteoarthritis is the most common form of arthritis that results in wrist joint pain. However, rheumatoid arthritis, posttraumatic arthritis, and psoriatic arthritis are also common causes of arthritic wrist pain. These types of arthritis can result in significant alteration in the biomechanics of the wrist because they affect not only the joint but also the tendons and other connective tissues that make up the functional unit.

SIGNS AND SYMPTOMS

Most patients presenting with wrist pain secondary to osteoarthritis or posttraumatic arthritis complain of pain that is localized around the wrist and hand. Activity makes the pain worse, whereas rest and heat provide some relief. The pain is constant and is characterized as aching; it may interfere with sleep. Some patients complain of a grating or popping sensation with use of the joint, and crepitus may be present on physical examination. If the pain and dysfunction are secondary to rheumatoid arthritis, the metacarpophalangeal joints are often involved, with characteristic deformity (Fig. 1.6).

In addition to pain, patients suffering from arthritis of the wrist joint often experience a gradual reduction in functional ability because of decreasing

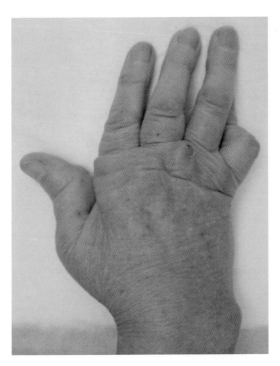

Fig. 1.6 Photograph of a rheumatoid hand; note ulnar axial deviation of the wrist. (From Trieb K. Treatment of the wrist in rheumatoid arthritis. *J Hand Surg.* 2008;33(1):113–123.)

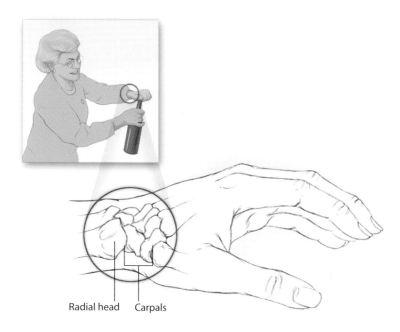

Radial head   Carpals

Fig. 1.7 Arthritis of the wrist often makes simple everyday tasks such as opening a bottle painful. (From Waldman S. *Atlas of Common Pain Syndromes*. 4th ed. Philadelphia: Elsevier; 2019 [Fig. 49-1]. 9780323547314.)

wrist range of motion that makes simple everyday tasks such as using a computer keyboard, holding a coffee cup, turning a doorknob, or unscrewing a bottle cap quite difficult (Fig. 1.7). With continued disuse, muscle wasting may occur, and adhesive capsulitis with subsequent ankylosis may develop. Dysfunction caused by arthritis of the wrist may result in tenosynovitis (Fig. 1.8).

TESTING

Plain radiographs are indicated in all patients who present with wrist pain (Fig. 1.9; also see Fig. 1.3). Based on the patient's clinical presentation, additional testing may be warranted, including a complete blood count, erythrocyte sedimentation rate, and antinuclear antibody testing. Magnetic resonance (MRI) and/or ultrasound imaging of the wrist is indicated if joint instability is thought to be present, as well as to further characterize the causes of pain and functional disability (Figs. 1.10, 1.11, and 1.12). If infection is suspected, Gram stain and culture of the synovial fluid should be performed on an emergency basis, and treatment with appropriate antibiotics should be started (Figs. 1.13 and 1.14).

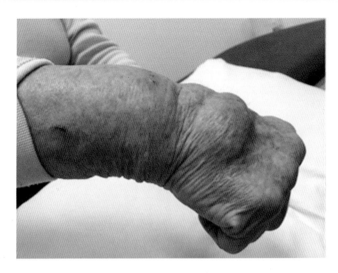

Fig. 1.8 Positive Tuck sign in a patient with severe extensor tenosynovitis of the wrist. Prominent 3 × 4 cm swelling over dorsum of hand with associated distal forearm swelling and intrinsic muscle wasting. (From Achilleos KM, Gaffney K. The Tuck sign-proliferative extensor tenosynovitis of the wrist. *Joint Bone Spine.* 2018 [Fig. 1a]. ISSN 1297-319X, https://doi.org/10.1016/j.jbspin.2018.11.007.)

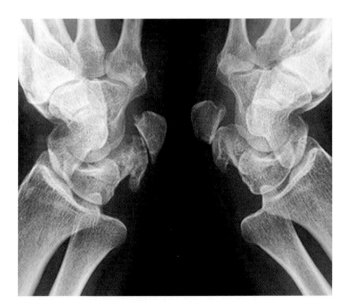

Fig. 1.9 Pisotriquetral joint osteoarthritis. Comparative ulnar side radiograph shows bilateral pisotriquetral joint osteoarthritis. (From Feydy A, Pluot E, Guerini H, Drapé J-L. Role of imaging in spine, hand, and wrist osteoarthritis. *Rheum Dis Clin North Am.* 2009:35(3):605−649)

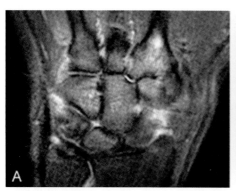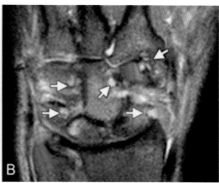

Fig. 1.10 Magnetic resonance imaging (MRI) may help identify arthritis of the wrist in patients with negative or equivocal x-rays. MRI scans of 51-year-old woman with early rheumatoid arthritis (RA) and normal x-ray finding at presentation. (A) Baseline coronal fat-suppressed T2-weighted image shows diffuse bone marrow edema with high signal intensity in carpal bones and base of second metacarpal bone. (B) At 18 months, follow-up, bone edema subsides with appearance of bone erosions *(arrows)* at sites of previous marrow edema. (From Dewan K, El-saadany H. Dynamic contrast enhanced MRI of wrist as a useful diagnostic tool in early rheumatoid arthritis. *Egypt J Radiol Nucl Med.* 2014;45(3): 803–810 [Fig. 4]. ISSN 0378-603X, https://doi.org/10.1016/j.ejrnm.2014.03.010, http://www.science-direct.com/science/article/pii/S0378603X14000564.)

DIFFERENTIAL DIAGNOSIS

The differential diagnosis of wrist pain is broad, and correct diagnosis will require use of the targeted history and physical examination combined with appropriate testing to drive diagnostic considerations (Table 1.1). Osteoarthritis is the most common form of arthritis that results in wrist joint pain. However, rheumatoid arthritis and posttraumatic arthritis are also common causes of wrist pain (see Fig. 1.6). Less common causes of arthritis-induced wrist pain include collagen vascular diseases, infection, villonodular synovitis, and Lyme disease. Acute infectious arthritis is usually accompanied by significant systemic symptoms, including fever and malaise, and should be easily recognized and treated with antibiotics (see Fig. 1.13). Collagen vascular diseases generally manifest as polyarthropathy rather than as monarthropathy limited to the wrist joint; however, wrist pain secondary to collagen vascular disease responds exceedingly well to the intraarticular injection technique described here.

TREATMENT

Initial treatment of the pain and functional disability associated with osteoarthritis of the wrist includes a combination of nonsteroidal antiinflammatory drugs (NSAIDs) or cyclooxygenase-2 inhibitors and physical therapy. Local

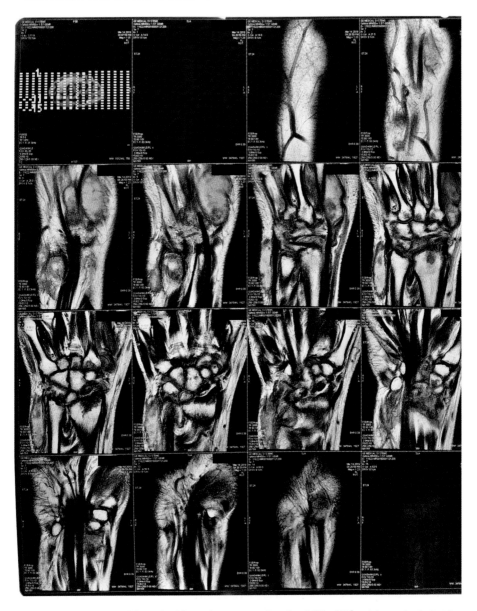

Fig. 1.11 Septic arthritis of the wrist. Magnetic resonance imaging (MRI) of the wrist reveals destruction of the radiocarpal joint, tenosynovitis changes of extensor carpi radialis brevis, and extensor digitorum tendons with mild subcutaneous soft tissue swelling suggestive of cellulitis, with fluid in the joint. (From Latief W, Asril E. Tuberculosis of the wrist mimicking rheumatoid arthritis—a rare case. *Int J Surg Case Rep*. 2019;63:13−18 [Fig. 3]. ISSN 2210-2612, https://doi.org/10.1016/j.ijscr.2019.08.023, http://www.sciencedirect.com/science/article/pii/S2210261219304869.)

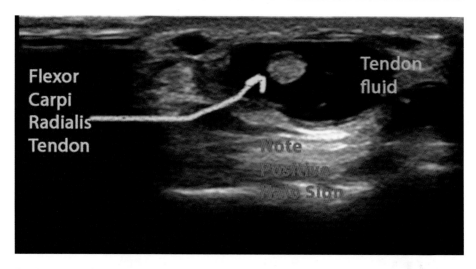

Fig. 1.12 Transverse ultrasound image demonstrating significant tendinitis of the flexor carpi radialis tendon. Not the positive halo sign secondary to effusion surrounding the inflamed tendon.

application of heat and cold may also be beneficial. Splinting the wrist in the neutral position may provide symptomatic relief and protect the joint from additional trauma. For patients who do not respond to these treatment modalities, intraarticular injection of local anesthetic and steroid is a reasonable next step (Fig. 1.15).

The injection of platelet-rich plasma and/or stem cells has been advocated to reduce the pain and functional disability of arthritis of the wrist.

Physical modalities, including local heat and gentle range-of-motion exercises, should be introduced several days after the patient begins treatment for arthritis of the wrist. Vigorous exercises should be avoided because they will exacerbate the patient's symptoms.

COMPLICATIONS AND PITFALLS

Joint protection is especially important in patients suffering from inflammatory arthritis of the wrist because repetitive trauma can result in further damage to the joint, tendons, and connective tissues. The major complication of intraarticular injection of the wrist is infection, although it should be exceedingly rare if strict aseptic technique is followed. The injection technique is safe if careful attention is paid to the clinically relevant anatomy; the ulnar nerve is especially susceptible to damage at the wrist. Approximately 25% of patients complain of a transient increase in pain after intraarticular injection of the wrist joint, and patients should be warned of this possibility.

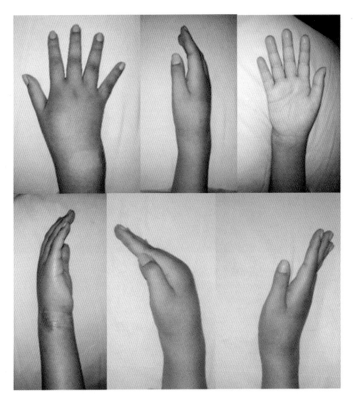

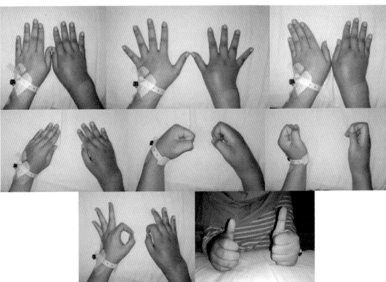

Fig. 1.13 Clinical appearance of septic arthritis of the wrist. (From Latief W, Asril E. Tuberculosis of the wrist mimicking rheumatoid arthritis—a rare case. *Int J Surg Case Rep.* 2019;63:13—18 [Fig. 1]. ISSN 2210-2612, https://doi.org/10.1016/j.ijscr.2019.08.023, http://www.sciencedirect.com/science/article/pii/S2210261219304869.)

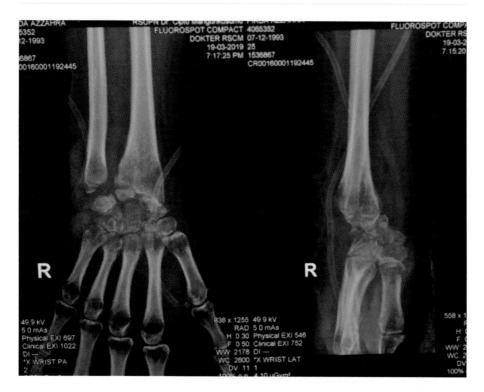

Fig. 1.14 Radiograph of the right wrist demonstrating diffuse demineralization and destruction of joint architecture in a patient with proven septic arthritis of the wrist. (From Latief W, Asril E. Tuberculosis of the wrist mimicking rheumatoid arthritis—a rare case. *Int J Surg Case Rep.* 2019;63:13–18 [Fig. 5]. ISSN 2210-2612, https://doi.org/10.1016/j.ijscr.2019.08.023, http://www.sciencedirect.com/science/article/pii/S2210261219304869.)

TABLE 1.1 ■ Causes of Wrist Pain

Bony Abnormalities

Fracture
Tumor
Osteomyelitis
Osteonecrosis
Kienböck disease and Preiser disease

Articular Abnormalities

Osteoarthritis
Rheumatoid arthritis

Collagen Vascular Diseases

Reiter syndrome
Psoriatic arthritis

(Continued)

TABLE 1.1 ■ **Causes of Wrist Pain—cont'd**

Crystal Deposition Diseases

Gout
Pseudogout
Pigmented villonodular synovitis
Sprain
Strain
Hemarthrosis

Periarticular Abnormalities

Tendon sheath disorders
Trigger finger
Flexor tenosynovitis
Extensor tenosynovitis
De Quervain tenosynovitis
Dupuytren contracture
Ganglion cyst
Gouty tophi
Subcutaneous nodules associated with rheumatoid arthritis
Glomus tumor

Neurologic Abnormalities

Median nerve entrapment
Carpal tunnel syndrome
Pronator syndrome
Anterior interosseous nerve syndrome
Ulnar nerve entrapment
Ulnar tunnel syndrome
Cubital tunnel syndrome
Cheiralgia paresthetica
Lower brachial plexus lesions
Cervical nerve root lesions
Spinal cord lesions
Syringomyelia
Spinal cord tumors
Reflex sympathetic dystrophy
Causalgia

Vascular Abnormalities

Vasculitis
Raynaud syndrome
Takayasu arteritis
Scleroderma

Referred Pain

Shoulder-hand syndrome
Angina

From Waldman S. *Physical Diagnosis of Pain: An Atlas of Signs and Symptoms.* 3rd ed. St. Louis: Elsevier; 2016 (table 102-10).

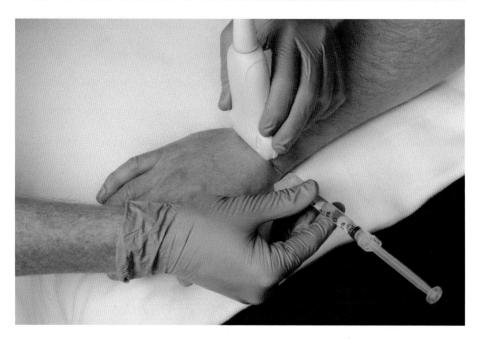

Fig. 1.15   Intraarticular injection of the wrist joint can serve as both a diagnostic and therapeutic maneuver.

HIGH-YIELD TAKEAWAYS

- The patient is afebrile, making an acute infectious etiology (e.g., septic arthritis) unlikely.
- The patient's symptomatology is not the result of acute trauma but more likely the result of repetitive microtrauma that has damaged the joint over time.
- The patient's pain is diffuse rather than highly localized as would be the case with a pathologic process such as fracture or de Quervain tenosynovitis.
- The patient's symptoms are unilateral and only involve one joint, which is more suggestive of a local process than a systemic polyarthropathy.
- Sleep disturbance is common and must be addressed concurrently with the patient's pain symptomatology.
- Plain radiographs will provide high-yield information regarding the bony contents of the joint, but ultrasound imaging and MRI will be more useful in identifying soft tissue pathology.

Suggested Readings

Bay COA, Willacy RA, Moses AR, et al. Nonspecific wrist pain in pediatric patients: a systematic review. *J Orthop*. 2020;22:308–315.

Brewer PE, Storey PA. The hand and wrist in rheumatoid and osteoarthritis. *Surg (Oxford)*. 2016;34(3):144—151.

Dineen HA, Greenberg JA. Ulnar-sided wrist pain in the athlete. *Clin Sport Med*. 2020;39(2):373—400.

Islam SU, Brown D, Cheung G. Management of osteoarthritis of the wrist and hand. *Orthop Trauma*. 2019;33(1):30—37.

Laulan J, Marteau E, Bacle G. Wrist osteoarthritis. *Orthop Traumatol Surg Res*. 2015;101(1): S1—S9.

Waldman SD. Abnormalities of the distal radioulnar joint. In: *Waldman's Comprehensive Atlas of Diagnostic Ultrasound of Painful Conditions*. Philadelphia, PA: Wolters Kluwer; 2016:353—360.

Waldman SD. Clinical correlates: functional anatomy of the wrist. In: *Physical Diagnosis of Pain: An Atlas of Signs and Symptoms*. 3rd ed. Philadelphia, PA: Saunders; 2016: 158—159.

Waldman SD. Intra-articular injection of the wrist joint. In: *Atlas of Pain Management Injection Techniques*. 4th ed. Philadelphia, PA: Elsevier; 2017:250—253.

Waldman SD, ed. Arthritis pain of the wrist. In: *Atlas of Common Pain Syndromes*. 4th ed. Philadelphia, PA: Saunders; 2019:190—194.

John Walker

A 30-Year-Old Male With Pain, Numbness, Weakness, and Paresthesias, Radiating Into the Thumb, Index and Middle Fingers

LEARNING OBJECTIVES

- Learn the common causes of wrist pain and hand pain.
- Learn the common causes of hand numbness.
- Develop an understanding of the unique relationship of the median nerve to the bones of the wrist.
- Develop an understanding of the anatomy of the median nerve.
- Develop an understanding of the causes of carpal tunnel syndrome.
- Develop an understanding of the differential diagnosis of carpal tunnel syndrome.
- Learn the clinical presentation of carpal tunnel syndrome.
- Learn how to examine the wrist.
- Learn how to examine the median nerve.
- Learn how to use physical examination to identify carpal tunnel syndrome.
- Develop an understanding of the treatment options for carpal tunnel syndrome.

John Walker

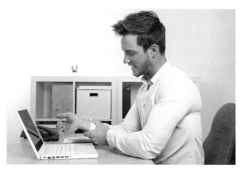

"Call me Johnny, everyone else does. You know, Johnny Walker? What the hell were my parents thinking? I never saw either of them take a drink!" I responded, "Okay, Johnny it is."

John Walker was a 30-year-old real estate agent with the chief complaint of "I have pain that goes from my wrist into my fingers, and my hand is weak." John stated that over the past several months, he began noticing a deep aching sensation in his hand and wrist, especially after using his laptop computer for long periods of time. The ache was associated with electric shock—like pains into the thumb, index finger, middle finger, and radial half of the ring finger. I asked John if he had experienced any numbness or weakness, and he replied, "Doc, it's funny that you asked. I am having trouble buttoning my top shirt button when I have to wear a tie, and lately I keep dropping my cell phone because I am having trouble holding it up to my ear. After a day at work, especially if I am using my laptop a lot, I have been noticing that my fingers, especially my thumb and index finger, have a pins-and-needles sensation." I asked John what he thought was causing his symptoms, and he said his wife thinks he has "the carpal tunnel. But, Doc, how smart could she be? She married me!" I responded, "John, she may actually be smarter than you think! Let me ask you a few more questions, then examine you so we can figure out if your wife is indeed correct."

I asked John what he had tried to make it better, and he said when he rested his hands and took a break from the laptop that seemed to make the pain better. After about 30 to 40 minutes the numbness got better. "Tylenol PM seems to help some, at least with the sleep," John reported. I asked John to describe any numbness he noticed associated with the pain, and he pointed to his right thumb and index finger. "Doc, most of the thumb and index finger are numb, and so is my middle finger." I asked John about any fever, chills, or other constitutional symptoms such as weight loss, night sweats, etc., and he shook his head no. He denied any antecedent wrist trauma, but noted that sometimes, if his hand wasn't positioned just right, he would get an electric shock—like pain that woke him up at night.

I asked John to point with one finger to show me where it hurt the most. He pointed to the middle of the dorsal wrist. He went on to say that he could live with the pain, but the electric shocks and numbness were "really bothering." He then asked, "Doc, could this have anything to do with diabetes?"

On physical examination, John was afebrile. His respirations were 18, his pulse was 74 and regular, and his blood pressure was 110/68. John's head, eyes, ears, nost, throat (HEENT) exam was normal, as was his cardiopulmonary exam. His thyroid was normal. His abdominal examination revealed no abnormal mass or organomegaly. There was no costovertebral angle (CVA) tenderness. There was no peripheral edema. His low back examination was unremarkable. Visual inspection of the right wrist was unremarkable. There was no rubor or color. There was no obvious infection or olecranon bursitis. There was a positive Tinel sign over the median nerve at the wrist (Fig. 2.1). I had Johnny fully flex both wrists and hold them in that position for 1 minute to see if I could elicit a positive Phalen test (Fig. 2.2). After about 45 seconds, Johnny began experiencing both pain and numbness. The left wrist examination was normal, but there was tenderness to palpation of the area over the carpal tunnel at the distal crease of the wrist. A careful neurologic examination of the upper extremities revealed decreased sensation in the distribution of the right median nerve as well as weakness of thumb

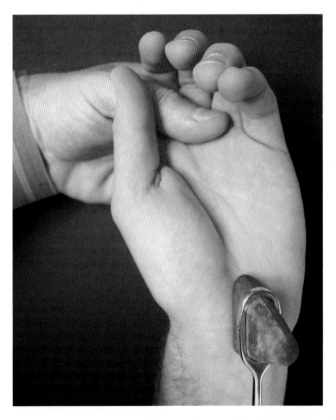

Fig. 2.1 Tinel sign for carpal tunnel syndrome. (From Waldman SD. *Physical Diagnosis of Pain: An atlas of signs and symptoms*. Philadelphia: Saunders; 2006:178.)

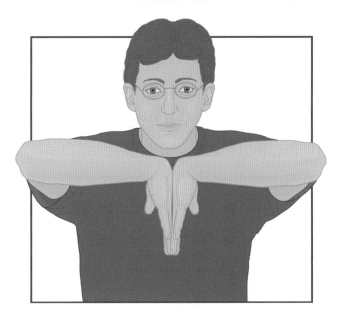

Fig. 2.2   A positive Phalen maneuver is highly indicative of carpal tunnel syndrome. (From Waldman SD. *Atlas of pain management injection techniques*. Philadelphia: Saunders; 2000.)

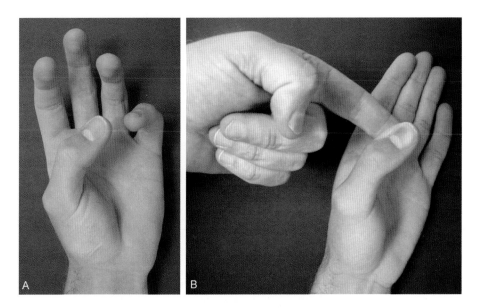

Fig. 2.3   The opponens weakness test for carpal tunnel syndrome. (A) The patient is asked to touch the tip of the little finger with the opposing thumb. (B) The clinician asked the patient to hold the thumb against the tip of the little finger. The clinician then tries to actively extend the thumb. Weakness suggests compromise of the median nerve. (From Waldman SD. *Physical diagnosis of pain: an atlas of signs and symptoms*. Philadelphia: Saunders; 2006:180.)

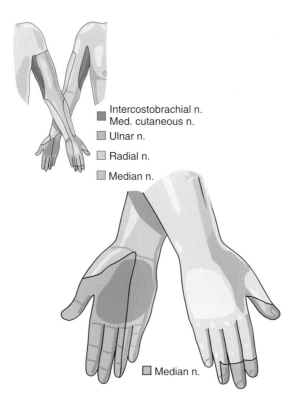

Intercostobrachial n.
Med. cutaneous n.
Ulnar n.
Radial n.
Median n.

Median n.

Fig. 2.4 Wasting of the thenar eminence is seen as carpal tunnel syndrome progresses. (From Waldman S. *Atlas of Interventional Pain Management.* 4th ed. Philadelphia, PA; Elsevier; 2015:267, [Fig. 59.7].)

opposition on the right as indicated by a positive opponens weakness test (Fig. 2.3). There was some wasting of the thenar eminence noted on the right (Fig. 2.4). I retorted, "Johnny, my friend, I think you have the carpal tunnel."

Key Clinical Points—What's Important and What's Not

THE HISTORY

- A history of the onset of right wrist pain with associated paresthesias and numbness radiating into the distribution of the median nerve
- Numbness of the thumb, index finger, and middle finger
- Weakness of opposition of the thumb
- No history of previous significant wrist pain
- Past medical history of diabetes
- No fever or chills

THE PHYSICAL EXAMINATION

- Patient is afebrile
- Positive Tinel sign at the wrist (see Fig. 2.1)
- Positive Phalen test (see Fig. 2.2)
- Positive opponens weakness test for carpal tunnel syndrome
- Weakness of the opposition of the thumb and index finger
- Numbness of the thumb, index, middle, and radial aspect of the ring finger in the distribution of the median nerve
- Wasting of the thenar eminence on the right (see Fig. 2.4)
- No evidence of infection

OTHER FINDINGS OF NOTE

- Normal HEENT examination
- Normal cardiovascular examination
- Normal pulmonary examination
- Normal abdominal examination
- No peripheral edema
- Normal left upper extremity neurologic examination, motor and sensory examination

 What Tests Would You Like to Order?

The following tests were ordered:
- Ultrasound of the right wrist
- Magnetic resonance imaging (MRI) of the right wrist
- Electromyography (EMG) and nerve conduction velocity testing of the right upper extremity

TEST RESULTS

Ultrasound examination of the right wrist at the distal wrist crease revealed a thickened and bulging transverse carpal ligament with a measurement of 0.8 mm. Enlargement of the median nerve with loss of the normal internal architecture was noted (Fig. 2.5).

MRI scan of the right wrist reveals fibrous synovial pannus and joint effusion (Fig. 2.6).

EMG and nerve conduction velocity testing revealed slowing of median nerve conduction across the wrist as well as denervation of the intrinsic muscles of the hand.

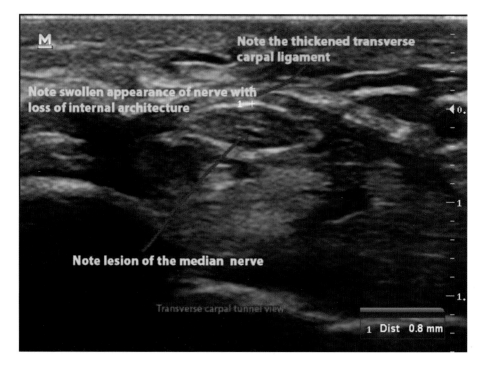

Fig. 2.5 Thickened and bulging transverse carpal ligament in patient with carpal tunnel syndrome. The transverse ligament measures 0.8 mm. Note the enlargement of the median nerve with loss of the normal internal architecture.

Clinical Correlation—Putting It All Together

What is the diagnosis?
- Carpal tunnel syndrome

The Science Behind the Diagnosis
ANATOMY

Carpal tunnel syndrome is caused by compression of the median nerve as it passes through the carpal canal at the wrist. The median nerve is made up of fibers from the C5-T1 spinal roots (Fig. 2.7). The nerve lies anterior and superior to the axillary artery in the 12-o'clock to 3-o'clock quadrant. Exiting the axilla, the median nerve descends into the upper arm along with the brachial artery. At the level of the elbow, the brachial artery is just medial to the biceps muscle. At this level, the median nerve lies just medial to the brachial artery. As the median nerve proceeds downward into the forearm, it gives off numerous branches that provide motor innervation to the flexor

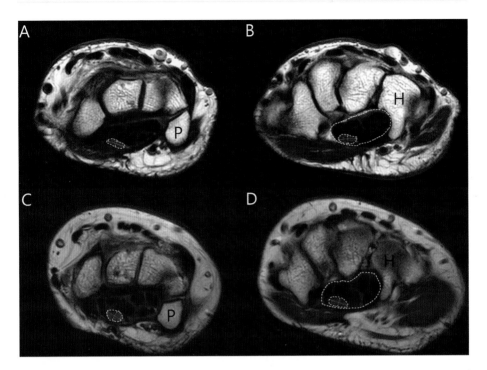

Fig. 2.6 Magnetic resonance imaging axial section of the wrist (T2-weighted sequence); carpal tunnel inlet (CTI) (A), carpal tunnel outlet (CTO) (B) of control patient and CTI (C), CTO (D) of patient with carpal tunnel syndrome. The area of margination with white dotted line indicates the cross-sectional area (CSA) of the entire carpal tunnel. The area of margination with yellow dotted line indicates the CSA of the median nerve. *H*, Hamate bone; *P*, pisiform. (From Park JS, Won H-C, Oh J-Y, et al. Value of cross-sectional area of median nerve by MRI in carpal tunnel syndrome. *Asian J Surg.* 2020;43(6):654−659 [Fig. 1]. ISSN 1015-9584, https://doi.org/10.1016/j.asjsur.2019.08.001, http://www.sciencedirect.com/science/article/pii/S1015958419301988.)

muscles of the forearm. These branches are susceptible to nerve entrapment by aberrant ligaments, muscle hypertrophy, and direct trauma. The nerve approaches the wrist overlying the radius. It lies deep to and between the tendons of the palmaris longus muscle and the flexor carpi radialis muscle at the wrist.

The median nerve then passes beneath the flexor retinaculum and through the carpal tunnel, with the nerve's terminal branches providing sensory innervation to a portion of the palmar surface of the hand as well as the palmar surface of the thumb, index and middle fingers, and radial portion of the ring finger (Figs. 2.8, 2.9, and 2.10). The median nerve also provides sensory innervation to the distal dorsal surface of the index and middle fingers and the radial portion of the ring finger. The carpal tunnel is bounded on three sides by the carpal bones and is covered by the transverse carpal ligament. In addition to the median nerve, it contains a number of flexor tendon sheaths, blood vessels, and lymphatics.

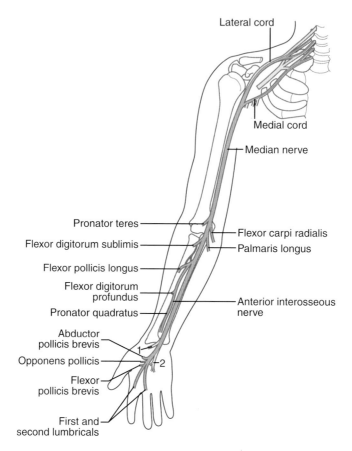

Fig. 2.7 The median nerve is made up of fibers from the C5-T1 spinal roots. The nerve lies anterior and superior to the axillary artery in the 12-o'clock to 3-o'clock quadrant. Exiting the axilla, the median nerve descends into the upper arm along with the brachial artery. At the level of the elbow, the brachial artery is just medial to the biceps muscle. At this level, the median nerve lies just medial to the brachial artery. As the median nerve proceeds downward into the forearm, it gives off numerous branches that provide motor innervation to the flexor muscles of the forearm. (From Preston DC, Shapiro BE, (eds.) Median neuropathy at the wrist. In: *Electromyography and Neuromuscular Disorders*. 3rd ed. London: Saunders; 2013:267–288.)

CLINICAL SYNDROME

Carpal tunnel syndrome is the most common entrapment neuropathy encountered in clinical practice. It is caused by compression of the median nerve as it passes through the carpal canal at the wrist. The most common causes of compression of the median nerve at this location include flexor tenosynovitis, rheumatoid arthritis, pregnancy, amyloidosis, and other space-occupying lesions that compromise the median nerve as it passes through this closed space. It occurs more commonly in women. This entrapment neuropathy presents as

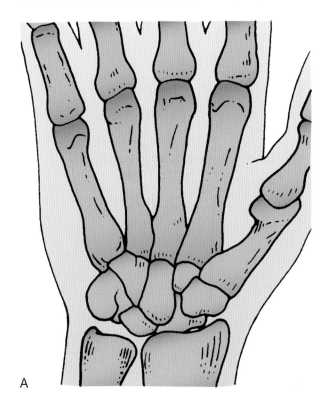

A

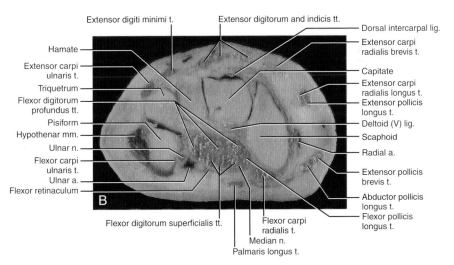

Extensor digiti minimi t.

Extensor digitorum and indicis tt.

Dorsal intercarpal lig.

Hamate

Extensor carpi radialis brevis t.

Extensor carpi ulnaris t.

Triquetrum

Capitate

Extensor carpi radialis longus t.

Flexor digitorum profundus tt.

Extensor pollicis longus t.

Pisiform

Deltoid (V) lig.

Hypothenar mm.

Scaphoid

Ulnar n.

Radial a.

Flexor carpi ulnaris t.

Ulnar a.

Extensor pollicis brevis t.

Flexor retinaculum

B

Abductor pollicis longus t.

Flexor pollicis longus t.

Flexor digitorum superficialis tt.

Flexor carpi radialis t.

Median n.

Palmaris longus t.

Fig. 2.8 Anatomy of the carpal tunnel. (A) Cross-sectional anatomy. (B) Cadaver section through carpal tunnel. Note the relationship of the median nerve to the flexor tendons. (From Kang HS, Resnick D, Ahn J. *MRI of the Extremities: An Anatomic Atlas*. 2nd ed. Philadelphia, PA: Saunders; 2002:177.)

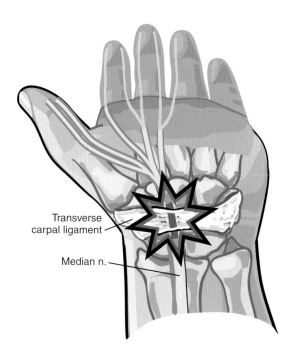

Transverse
carpal ligament

Median n.

Fig. 2.9 Carpal tunnel syndrome: clinically relevant anatomy. (From Waldman S. *Physical Diagnosis of Pain: An Atlas of Signs and Symptoms*. 4th ed. Philadelphia: Elsevier; 2021 [Fig. 121-1].)

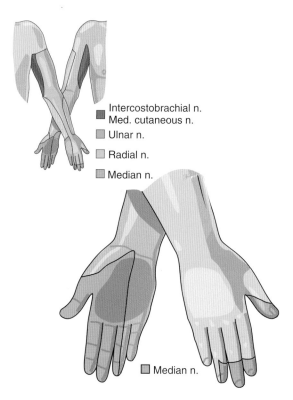

Intercostobrachial n.
Med. cutaneous n.
Ulnar n.
Radial n.
Median n.

Median n.

Fig. 2.10 Sensory distribution of the median nerve. (From Waldman S. *Atlas of Interventional Pain Management*. 5th ed. Philadelphia: Elsevier; 2021 [Fig. 61-7].)

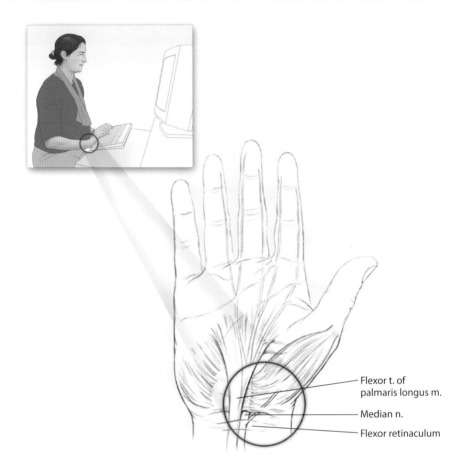

Flexor t. of
palmaris longus m.

Median n.

Flexor retinaculum

Fig. 2.11 Poor positioning of the hand and wrist during keyboarding can result in carpal tunnel syndrome. (From Waldman S. *Atlas of Common Pain Syndromes*. 4th ed. Philadelphia: Elsevier; 2019 [Fig. 50-1]. 9780323547314.)

pain, numbness, paresthesias, and associated weakness in the hand and wrist that radiate to the thumb, index finger, middle finger, and radial half of the ring finger. These symptoms may also radiate proximal to the entrapment into the forearm. Untreated, progressive motor deficit and, ultimately, flexion contracture of the affected fingers can result. Symptoms usually begin after repetitive wrist motions or repeated pressure on the wrist, such as resting the wrists on the edge of a computer keyboard (Fig. 2.11; Box 2.1). Direct trauma to the median nerve as it enters the carpal tunnel may result in a similar clinical presentation. Recent studies have suggested a higher incidence of abnormalities of connective tissue coding genes in patients suffering from carpal tunnel syndrome when compared with normal controls.

BOX 2.1 ■ Conditions Associated With Carpal Tunnel Syndrome

Structural/Anatomic
- Lipoma
- Ganglion
- Neuroma
- Aneurysm
- Acromegaly
- Fracture

Inflammatory
- Tenosynovitis
- Collagen vascular disease
  - Rheumatoid arthritis
  - Scleroderma
- Gout

Neuropathic/Ischemic
- Diabetes
- Alcoholism
- Vitamin abnormalities
- Ischemic neuropathies
- Peripheral neuropathies
- Amyloidosis

Shifts in Fluid Balance
- Pregnancy
- Hypothyroidism
- Obesity
- Kidney failure
- Menopause

Repetitive Stress Related
- Abnormal hand and wrist position
- Excessive flexion
- Microtrauma
- Vibration

SIGNS AND SYMPTOMS

Physical findings include tenderness over the median nerve at the wrist. A positive Tinel sign is usually present over the median nerve as it passes beneath the flexor retinaculum (see Fig. 2.1). A positive Phalen maneuver is highly suggestive of carpal tunnel syndrome. The Phalen maneuver is performed by having the patient place the wrists in complete unforced flexion for at least 30 seconds (see Fig. 2.2). If the median nerve is entrapped at the wrist, this maneuver reproduces the symptoms of carpal tunnel syndrome. Weakness of thumb opposition and wasting of the thenar eminence are often seen in advanced cases of carpal tunnel syndrome; however, because of the complex motion of the thumb, subtle motor deficits can easily be missed (see Figs. 2.3 and 2.4). Early in the course of carpal tunnel syndrome, the only physical finding other than tenderness over the median nerve may be the loss of sensation in the foregoing fingers.

TESTING

Electromyography can distinguish cervical radiculopathy and diabetic polyneuropathy from carpal tunnel syndrome. Plain radiographs are indicated in all patients who present with carpal tunnel syndrome, to rule out occult bony disorders. Based on the patient's clinical presentation, additional testing may be warranted, including a complete blood count, uric acid level, erythrocyte sedimentation rate, and antinuclear antibody testing. MRI of the wrist is indicated if joint instability or a space-occupying lesion is suspected or to confirm the actual cause of median nerve compression (Fig. 2.12; also see Fig. 2.6). Ultrasound imaging may be useful in the evaluation of the median nerve as it passes through the carpal tunnel (see Fig. 2.7). Studies have suggested a strong correlation between the cross-sectional area of the nerve and clinical carpal tunnel syndrome (Fig. 2.13). Injection of the median nerve at the carpal tunnel with local anesthetic and/or steroid may serve as both a diagnostic and therapeutic maneuver (Fig. 2.14).

DIFFERENTIAL DIAGNOSIS

Median nerve entrapment at the wrist is often misdiagnosed as golfer's wrist and this fact accounts for the many patients whose "golfer's wrist"

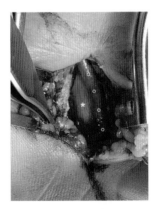

Fig. 2.12 Intraoperative image of a large persistent median artery (open circles) compressing the ventral surface of the median nerve (asterisk) and in the line of incision. (From Shields L., Vasudeva GI, Zhang Y, Shields C. Acute carpal tunnel syndrome: Clinical, electromyographic, and ultrasound features in 25 patients. *Clinical Neurology and Neurosurgery*. 2021;210:106984 [Fig. 4].)

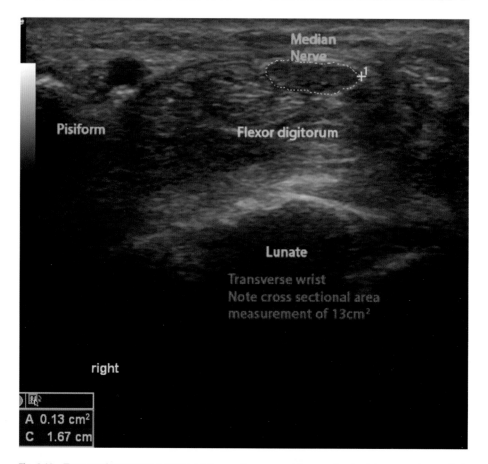

Fig. 2.13 Transverse ultrasound image of the median nerve at the proximal wrist crease demonstrating an increased cross-sectional area of the 13 cm², which is highly suggestive of carpal tunnel syndrome. Note the loss of the normal neural echotexture of the median nerve.

fails to respond to conservative measures. Cubital tunnel syndrome can be distinguished from golfer's wrist in that in cubital tunnel syndrome, the maximal tenderness to palpation is over the median nerve 1 inch below the medial epicondyle, whereas with golfer's wrist, the maximal tenderness to palpation is directly over the medial epicondyle. Cubital tunnel syndrome should also be differentiated from cervical radiculopathy involving the C7 or C8 roots and golfer's wrist. It should be remembered that cervical radiculopathy and median nerve entrapment may coexist as the so-called "double crush" syndrome. The double crush syndrome is seen most commonly with median nerve entrapment at the wrist or carpal tunnel syndrome.

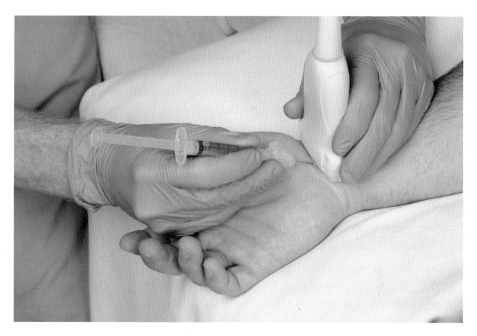

Fig. 2.14 Proper needle placement for ultrasound-guided injection for carpal tunnel syndrome utilizing an out-of-plane approach at the wrist.

TREATMENT

A short course of conservative therapy consisting of simple analgesics, nonsteroidal antiinflammatory agents, or COX-2 inhibitors, and splinting to avoid wrist flexion is indicated in patients who present with median nerve entrapment at the wrist. If the patient does not experience a marked improvement in symptoms within 1 week, careful injection of the median nerve at the wrist using the following technique is a reasonable next step.

Median nerve injection at the wrist is carried out by placing the patient in the supine position with the arm fully adducted at the patient's side and the wrist slightly flexed with the dorsum of the hand resting on a folded towel. A total of 5 to 7 mL of local anesthetic is drawn up in a 12-mL sterile syringe. A total of 80 mg of depot steroid is added to the local anesthetic with the first block and 40 mg of depot steroid is added with subsequent blocks.

The clinician then identifies the olecranon process and the medial epicondyle of the humerus. The median nerve sulcus between these two bony landmarks is then identified. After preparation of the skin with antiseptic solution, a 5/8-inch, 25-gauge needle is inserted just proximal to the sulcus and is slowly advanced in a slightly cephalad trajectory. As the needle advances approximately ½ inch, a strong paresthesia in the distribution of the median nerve will be elicited. The patient should be warned that a paresthesia will occur and to say "there!!!!" as soon as the paresthesia is felt. After paresthesia is elicited and its distribution identified, gentle aspiration is carried out to identify blood. If the aspiration test is negative and no persistent paresthesia into the distribution of the median nerve remains, 5 to 7 mL of solution is slowly injected, with the patient being monitored closely for signs of local anesthetic toxicity. If no paresthesia can be elicited, a similar amount of solution is slowly injected in a fan-like manner just proximal to the notch with care being taken to avoid intravascular injection. Ultrasound guided injection may be useful to decrease the incidence of needle-induced complications.

HIGH-YIELD TAKEAWAYS

- The patient is afebrile, making an acute infectious etiology unlikely.
- The patient's symptomatology is thought to be the result of prolonged pressure on the right median nerve at the wrist.
- Physical examination and testing should be focused on the identification of the various causes of carpal tunnel syndrome.
- The patient exhibits the neurologic and physical examination findings that are highly suggestive of carpal tunnel syndrome.
- The patient's symptoms are unilateral, suggestive of a local process rather than a systemic inflammatory process.
- Plain radiographs will provide high-yield information regarding the bony contents of the joint, but ultrasound imaging and MRI will be more useful in identifying soft tissue pathology that may be responsible for median nerve compromise at the wrist.
- EMG and nerve conduction velocity testing will help delineate the location and degree of nerve compromise if median nerve compromise is suspected.

Suggested Readings

Borire AA, Hughes AR, Lueck CJ, et al. Sonographic differences in carpal tunnel syndrome with normal and abnormal nerve conduction studies. *J Clin Neurosci.* 2016;34:77−80.

Csillik A, Bereczki D, Bora L, et al. The significance of ultrasonographic carpal tunnel outlet measurements in the diagnosis of carpal tunnel syndrome. *Clin Neurophysiol.* 2016;127(12):3516−3523.

Raissi GR, Ghazaei F, Forogh B, et al. The effectiveness of radial extracorporeal shock waves for treatment of carpal tunnel syndrome: a randomized clinical trial. *Ultrasound Med Biol.* 2017;43(2):453−460.

Waldman SD. Carpal tunnel syndrome. In: *Pain Review.* 2nd ed. Philadelphia: Elsevier; 2017:259−260.

Waldman SD. Carpal tunnel syndrome and other disorders of the median nerve at the wrist. In: *Waldman's Comprehensive Atlas of Diagnostic Ultrasound of Painful Conditions.* Philadelphia: Wolters Kluwer; 2016:370–385.

Waldman SD. Injection technique for carpal tunnel syndrome. In: *Atlas of Pain Management Injection Techniques.* 4th ed. Philadelphia: Elsevier; 2017:269–273.

Waldman SD, Campbell RSD. Carpal tunnel syndrome. In: *Imaging of Pain.* Philadelphia: Saunders; 2011:319–321.

Chase Armstrong

A 32-Year-Old Male With Pain and Electric Shock–Like Sensation Radiating Into the Lateral Forearm and Ring and Little Fingers

LEARNING OBJECTIVES

- Learn the common causes of wrist and hand pain.
- Learn the common causes of hand numbness.
- Develop an understanding of the unique relationship of the ulnar nerve to the ulnar artery and the ligaments and bones of the wrist.
- Develop an understanding of the anatomy of the ulnar nerve and the Guyon canal.
- Develop an understanding of the causes of ulnar nerve entrapment at the wrist.
- Develop an understanding of the differential diagnosis of ulnar nerve entrapment at the wrist.
- Learn the clinical presentation of ulnar nerve entrapment at the wrist.
- Learn how to examine the wrist.
- Learn how to examine the ulnar nerve.
- Learn how to use physical examination to identify ulnar nerve entrapment at the wrist.
- Develop an understanding of the treatment options for ulnar nerve entrapment at the wrist.

Chase Armstrong

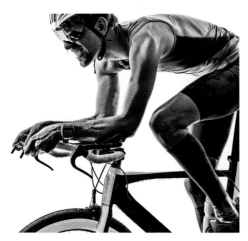

Chase Armstrong is a 32-year-old cycling enthusiast who I had been taking care of for the last several years. I last saw him for a hamstring strain following an ultra-endurance cycling event. His chief complaint today is "I have pain and numbness in my little finger and the outside of my ring finger." Chase stated that over the past several months, in addition to the numbness, he began noticing a deep aching sensation in his wrist and hand. It was associated with electric shock–like pains into the ring and little fingers on the right, especially when he rode for long distances. "At first, I thought it was my seat height, so I adjusted it, but that didn't do anything but give me a backache. So, then I thought it was the handlebars, but that wasn't it either."

I asked Chase if he had experienced any other symptoms, and he replied, "Doc, it's funny that you asked, as I am having the hardest time getting my keys out of my pants pocket because my little finger keeps catching on the edge of the pocket. And after a day at work, I have begun noticing that my little finger and part of my right ring finger, the part next to my little finger, are numb!" (Fig. 3.1) I asked Chase what he thought was causing his symptoms, but he had no idea. He was an iron man, and nothing ever slowed him down. I asked what he had tried to make it better, and he reported using a heating pad on his wrist at night, which "seemed to make the pain better, but the numbness worse. Tylenol PM seemed to help some, at least with sleep." I asked Chase to describe any numbness he noticed associated with the pain, and he pointed to his right little finger and the ulnar aspect of his ring finger. "Doc, the whole little finger is numb, but just part of my ring finger goes to sleep. The pins-and-needles sensation drives me crazy!" I asked Chase about any fever, chills, or other constitutional symptoms such as weight loss, night sweats, etc., and he shook his head no. He denied any antecedent wrist trauma, but noted that sometimes the electric shock–like pain woke him up at night.

I asked Chase to point with one finger to show me where it hurt the most. He pointed to the ulnar aspect of the right wrist. He went on to say that he could live with the pain, "but the crazy way my fingers are acting kind of scares me. I have to be able to hold the handlebars." He then asked, "Doc, my partner keeps insisting that all of this is from my cycling. That seems silly to me; I'd love to know what you think." I said that the cycling could certainly be a factor in his pain, weakness, and numbness, but that remained to be seen.

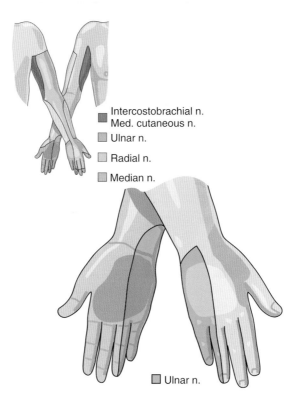

Intercostobrachial n.
Med. cutaneous n.
Ulnar n.
Radial n.
Median n.

Ulnar n.

Fig. 3.1 Sensory distribution of the ulnar nerve. (From Waldman S. *Atlas of Interventional Pain Management*. 5th ed. Philadelphia: Elsevier; 2021 [Fig. 62-6].)

On physical examination, Chase was afebrile. His respirations were 16, his pulse was 64 and regular, and his blood pressure was 110/68. Chase's head, eyes, ears, nose, throat (HEENT) exam was normal, as was his cardiopulmonary exam. His thyroid was normal. His abdominal examination revealed no abnormal mass or organomegaly. There was no costovertebral angle (CVA) tenderness. There was no peripheral edema. His low back examination was unremarkable. Visual inspection of the right wrist was unremarkable. There was no ecchymosis, rubor, or color and there was no obvious infection. There was a positive Tinel sign over the right ulnar nerve at the wrist. Examination of Chase's hands revealed no stigmata of osteoarthritis or rheumatoid arthritis. The left wrist examination was normal, but there was mild crepitus on passive flexion and extension of his right wrist. A careful neurologic examination of the upper extremities revealed decreased sensation in the distribution of the distal ulnar nerve as well as weakness of the intrinsic muscles of the right hand and weakness to the adductor pollicis brevis and flexor pollicis brevis (Fig. 3.2). Deep tendon reflexes were normal. Chase exhibited a positive Froment sign as well as a little finger adduction sign (Fig. 3.3). Jeanne sign was also positive (Fig. 3.4).

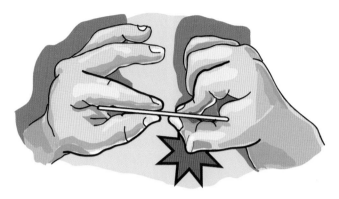

Fig. 3.2   Froment sign is elicited by asking the patient to grasp a piece of paper lightly between the thumb and index finger of each hand and monitoring flexion of the thumb interphalangeal joint on the affected side. (From Waldman S. *Atlas of Common Pain Syndromes*. 4th ed. Philadelphia: Elsevier; 2019 [Fig. 45-2 A].)

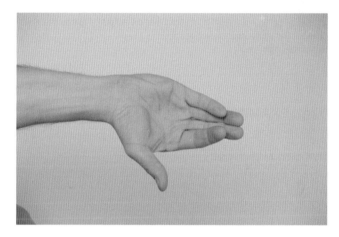

Fig. 3.3   The little finger adduction test evaluates the strength in the interosseous muscles of the hand that are innervated by the ulnar nerve. It is performed by asking the patient to touch the little finger to the index finger. (From Waldman SD. The little finger adduction test for ulnar nerve entrapment at the elbow. In: *Physical Diagnosis of Pain: An Atlas of Signs and Symptoms*. 2nd ed. Philadelphia: Saunders; 2010:126,128.)

Key Clinical Points—What's Important and What's Not

THE HISTORY

- A history of the onset of right wrist and hand pain with associated paresthesias into the distribution of the ulnar nerve
- Numbness of the little finger and ulnar aspect of the ring finger on the right
- Hand weakness
- No history of previous significant wrist pain
- No fever or chills

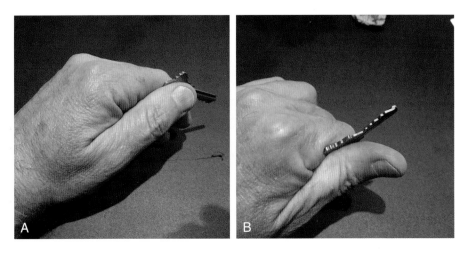

Fig. 3.4 (A) The Jeanne test is performed by asking the patient to lightly grasp a key between the thumb and radial aspect of the index finger of each hand and monitoring the flexion of the thumb inter-phalangeal joint on the affected side. (B) The patient is then asked to grasp the key more tightly. The Jeanne test is positive if the metacarpophalangeal joint of the affected thumb hyperextends to stabilize the joint to increase grasp pressure.

THE PHYSICAL EXAMINATION

- Patient is afebrile
- Positive Tinel sign at the wrist
- Positive Jeanne, Froment, and little finger adduction test (see Figs. 3.2, 3.3, and 3.4)
- Weakness of the intrinsic muscles of the right hand
- Numbness of the little and ring fingers in the distribution of the ulnar nerve (see Fig. 3.1)
- Hand findings suggestive of rheumatoid arthritis, including mild synovitis and ulnar drift
- No evidence of infection

OTHER FINDINGS OF NOTE

- Normal HEENT examination
- Normal cardiovascular examination
- Normal pulmonary examination
- Normal abdominal examination
- No peripheral edema
- Normal left upper extremity neurologic examination, motor and sensory examination

What Tests Would You Like to Order?

The following tests were ordered:
- Ultrasound of the right wrist
- Magnetic resonance imaging (MRI) of the right wrist
- Electromyography (EMG) and nerve conduction velocity testing of the right upper extremity

TEST RESULTS

Ultrasound examination of the right wrist revealed flattening and enlargement of the ulnar nerve at the level of the ulnar tunnel. The cross-sectional area of the ulnar nerve was 0.10 cm^2 (Fig. 3.5).

MRI scan of the right wrist revealed a ganglion cyst compressing the ulnar nerve and vessels at the ulnar tunnel (Fig. 3.6).

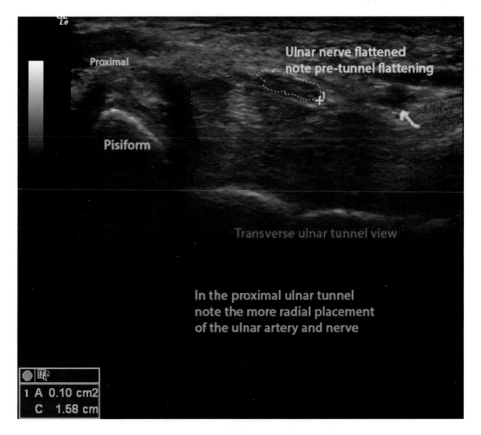

Fig. 3.5   Transverse ultrasound view of the ulnar nerve at the level of the ulnar tunnel. Note the flattening and enlargement of the nerve. The cross-sectional area is 0.10 cm^2.

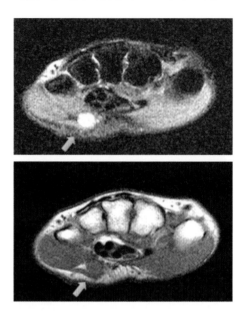

Fig. 3.6 Preoperative MRI displayed an intraneural ganglion cyst related to the ulnar nerve (From UfukÖztürk, AhmetSalduz, Mehmet Demire, TunaPehlivanoğlu, Sevan Sivacioğlu. Intraneural ganglion cyst of the ulnar nerve in an unusual location: a case report. *International Journal of Surgery Case Reports*. 2017;31:61−64 [Fig. 1].)

EMG and nerve conduction velocity testing revealed slowing of ulnar nerve conduction across the wrist as well as denervation of the intrinsic muscles of the hand.

Clinical Correlation—Putting It All Together

What is the diagnosis?
- Ulnar tunnel syndrome

The Science Behind the Diagnosis

ANATOMY

Arising from fibers from the C8-T1 nerve roots of the medial cord of the brachial plexus, the ulnar nerve lies anterior and inferior to the axillary artery in the 3-o'clock to 6-o'clock quadrant as it passes through the axilla. As the ulnar nerve exits the axilla, it passes inferiorly adjacent to the brachial artery. At the middle of the upper arm, the ulnar nerve turns medially to pass between the olecranon process and medial epicondyle of the humerus (Fig. 3.7). Continuing its downward path, the ulnar nerve passes between the heads of the flexor carpi ulnaris moving radially along with the ulnar artery. At a point approximately 1 inch proximal to the crease of the wrist, the ulnar nerve divides into the dorsal

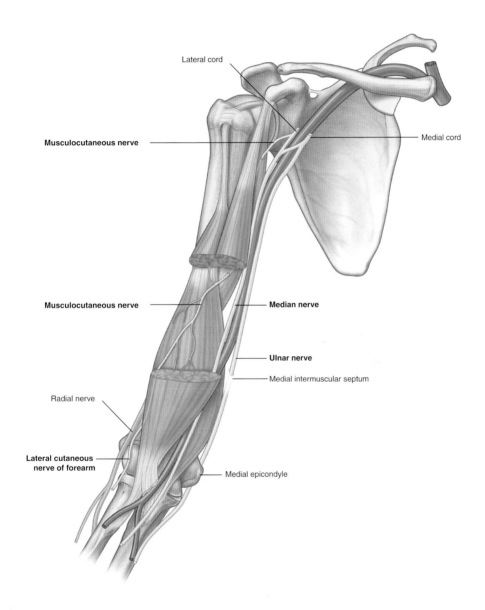

Fig. 3.7 Anatomy of the ulnar nerve. (From Drake R, Vogl W, Mitchell A. *Gray's Anatomy for Students*. 4th ed. Philadelphia: Churchill Livingstone; 2020 [Fig. 7-68].)

and palmar branches. The dorsal branch provides sensation to the ulnar aspect of the dorsum of the hand and the dorsal aspect of the little finger and the ulnar half of the ring finger (see Fig. 3.1). The palmar branch provides sensory innervation to the ulnar aspect of the palm of the hand and the palmar aspect of the little finger and the ulnar half of the ring finger. The ulnar nerve then enters the palm of the hand via Guyon canal (Fig. 3.8).

In contradistinction to the median nerve, which passes beneath the flexor retinaculum, the ulnar nerve and artery lie above the flexor retinaculum. The nerve then gives off its terminal branches, the superficial and deep branches of the ulnar nerve (Fig. 3.9). The superficial branch provides motor innervation to the palmaris brevis muscle and sensory innervation to the ulnar aspect of the hand (Fig. 3.10). The deep branch of ulnar nerve provides motor innervation to the hypothenar muscles, the third and fourth lumbricals, all of the interosseous muscles, the adductor pollicis muscle, and the deep head of the flexor pollicis brevis muscle. The deep branch of the ulnar nerve also provides sensory innervation to the wrist joint.

CLINICAL SYNDROME

Ulnar tunnel syndrome is an entrapment neuropathy of the ulnar nerve characterized by pain, numbness, and paresthesias of the wrist that radiate into the ulnar aspect of the palm and dorsum of the hand and the little finger and the ulnar half of the ring finger. These symptoms also may radiate proximal to the nerve entrapment into the forearm. The pain of ulnar tunnel syndrome is often described as aching or burning, with associated pins-and-needles paresthesias.

Similar to carpal tunnel syndrome, ulnar tunnel syndrome occurs more commonly in women than in men. Also similar to carpal tunnel syndrome, the pain of ulnar tunnel syndrome is frequently worse at night and worsened by vigorous flexion and extension of the wrist. The onset of symptoms usually follows repetitive wrist motions; direct trauma to the wrist, such as wrist fractures; direct trauma to the proximal hypothenar eminence, such as may occur when the hand is used to hammer on hubcaps; or from handlebar compression during long-distance cycling. Ulnar tunnel syndrome also is seen in patients with rapid weight gain, rheumatoid arthritis, Dupuytren disease, or during pregnancy. Untreated, progressive motor deficit and ultimately flexion contracture of the affected fingers can result.

Ulnar tunnel syndrome is caused by compression of the ulnar nerve as it passes through Guyon canal at the wrist (see Fig. 3.8). The most common causes of compression of the ulnar nerve at this anatomic location include space-occupying lesions, such as ganglion cysts and ulnar artery aneurysms; fractures of the distal ulna and carpals; trauma to the ulnar nerve; and repetitive motion

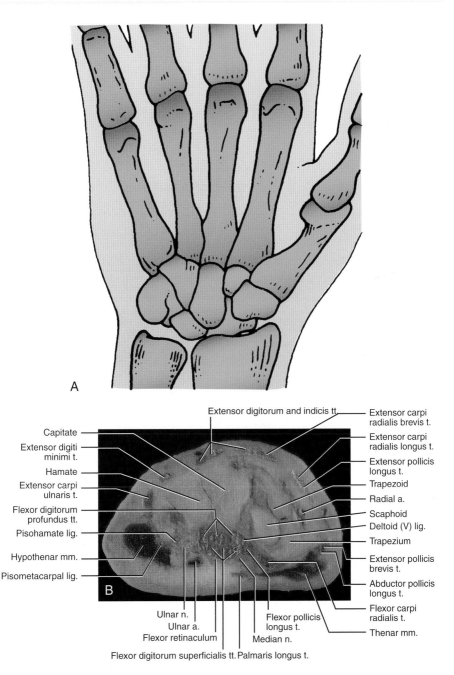

Fig. 3.8 Anatomic section demonstrating Guyon canal. (A) Anatomic Drawing. (B) Cadaver cross-sectional anatomy. (A, From Kang HS, Resnick D, Ahn J. *MRI of the Extremities: An Anatomic Atlas*. 2nd ed. Philadelphia: Saunders; 2002; B, From Kang HS, Resnick D, Ahn J. *MRI of the Extremities: An Anatomic Atlas*. 2nd ed. Philadelphia, PA: Saunders; 2002:178.)

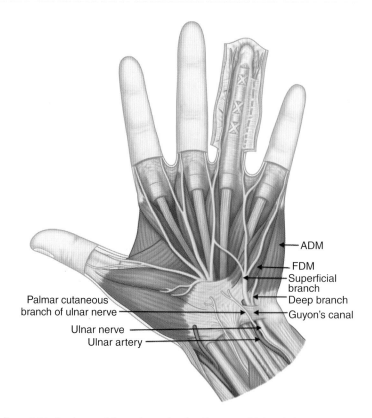

Fig. 3.9 Superficial structures of the palm and wrist. The superficial and deep branches of the ulnar nerve are indicated. *ADM*, Abductor digiti minimi; *FDM*, flexor digiti minimi. (From Bachoura A, Jacoby SM. Ulnar tunnel syndrome. *Orthop Clin North Am.* 2012;43(4):467–474; Waldman S. *Atlas of Interventional Pain Management.* 5th ed. Philadelphia: Elsevier; 2021 [Fig. 62.4].)

injuries that compromise the ulnar nerve as it passes through this closed space (Fig. 3.11). This entrapment neuropathy manifests most commonly as a pure motor neuropathy without pain, which is due to compression of the deep palmar branch of the ulnar nerve as it passes through Guyon canal. This pure motor neuropathy manifests as painless paralysis of the intrinsic muscles of the hand. Ulnar tunnel syndrome also may manifest as a mixed sensory and motor neuropathy. Clinically, this mixed neuropathy manifests as pain and the previously described motor deficits.

SIGNS AND SYMPTOMS

Physical findings include tenderness over the ulnar nerve at the wrist. A positive Tinel sign over the ulnar nerve as it passes beneath the transverse carpal ligament is usually present. If the sensory branches are involved, decreased

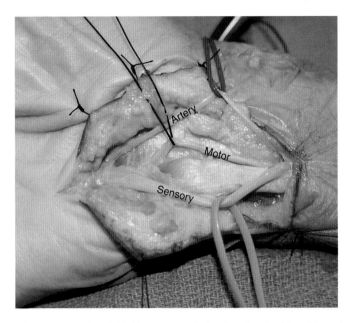

Fig. 3.10 The ulnar nerve can be divided into sensory (palmar) and motor (dorsal) branches. Note the fibrous arch of the hypothenar muscles under which the deep motor branch passes on its way out of the ulnar tunnel. The ulnar artery travels along the radial side of the nerve through the tunnel, after which it splits and becomes the deep and superficial palmar arches. *(Blue tag)* Sensory branch; *(black tag)* motor branch; *(red tag)* ulnar artery. (From Waugh RP, Pellegrini Jr VD. Ulnar tunnel syndrome. *Hand Clin.* 2007;23:301–310; Waldman S. *Atlas of Uncommon Pain Syndromes.* 4th ed. Philadelphia: Elsevier; 2020 [Fig. 50-1].)

sensation occurs into the ulnar aspect of the hand and the little finger and the ulnar half of the ring finger. Depending on the location of neural compromise, the patient may have weakness of the intrinsic muscles of the hand as evidenced by the inability to spread the fingers, weakness of the hypothenar eminence, or both (Figs. 3.12 and 3.13). If left untreated, the patient suffering from ulnar tunnel syndrome may develop wasting of the intrinsic muscles of the hand (see Fig. 3.13).

TESTING

EMG helps distinguish cervical radiculopathy, diabetic polyneuropathy, and Pancoast tumor from ulnar tunnel syndrome. Plain radiographs are indicated in all patients who present with ulnar tunnel syndrome to rule out occult bony pathologic processes. Based on the patient's clinical presentation, additional tests, including complete blood cell count, uric acid level, erythrocyte sedimentation rate, and antinuclear antibody testing, may be indicated. MRI and ultrasound imaging of the wrist are indicated to help confirm the diagnosis and

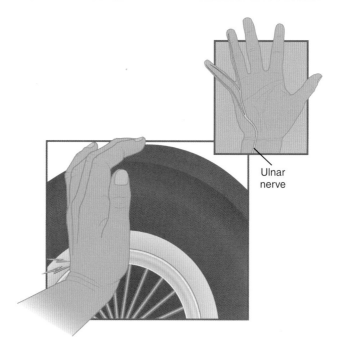

Fig. 3.11   The most common causes of compression of the ulnar nerve at the wrist includes space-occupying lesions, such as ganglion cysts and ulnar artery aneurysms; fractures of the distal ulna and carpals; trauma to the ulnar nerve; and repetitive motion injuries that compromise the ulnar nerve as it passes through this closed space. (From Waldman SD. *Atlas of Pain Management Injection Techniques*. Philadelphia, PA: Saunders; 2000:151.)

whether joint instability, trauma, or a space-occupying lesion is the cause of the patient's neurologic findings (Figs. 3.14 and 3.15; see also Figs. 3.5 and 3.6). Injection of the ulnar nerve as it passes through the ulnar tunnel with local anesthetic and/or steroid technique can serve as a diagnostic and therapeutic maneuver (Fig. 3.16). Ultrasound and color Doppler guidance will improve the accuracy of needle placement and decrease the incidence of needle-induced complications (Figs. 3.17 and 3.18).

DIFFERENTIAL DIAGNOSIS

Ulnar tunnel syndrome often is misdiagnosed as arthritis of the carpometacarpal joints, cervical radiculopathy, Pancoast tumor, and diabetic neuropathy (Fig. 3.19). Patients with arthritis of the carpometacarpal joint usually have radiographic evidence and physical findings suggestive of arthritis. Most patients with a cervical radiculopathy have reflex, motor, and sensory changes associated with neck pain, whereas patients with ulnar tunnel syndrome have

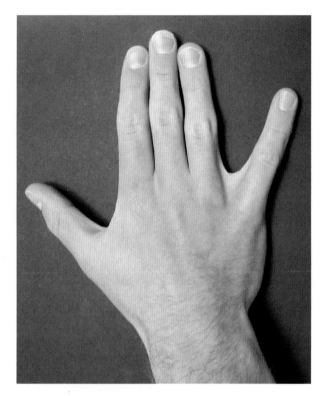

Fig. 3.12 The spread sign for ulnar tunnel syndrome. (From Waldman S. *Physical Diagnosis of Pain: An Atlas of Signs and Symptoms*. 4th ed. Philadelphia: Elsevier; 2021 [Fig. 128-4].)

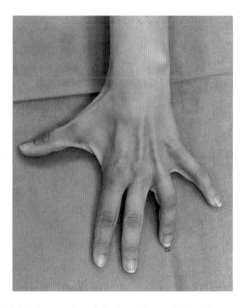

Fig. 3.13 Wasting of the intrinsic muscles of the hand in a patient with sever ulnar nerve entrapment at the wrist. (From Lauretti L, D'Alessandris QG, De Simone C, et al. Ulnar nerve entrapment at the wrist. A surgical series and a systematic review of the literature. *J Clin Neurosci*. 2017;46:99-108 [Fig. 2]. ISSN 0967-5868, https://doi.org/10.1016/j.jocn.2017.08.012, http://www.sciencedirect.com/science/article/pii/S0967586817309098.)

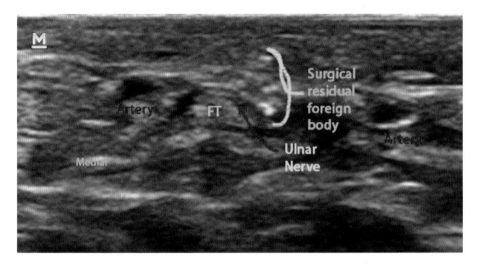

Fig. 3.14 Ultrasound image demonstrating retained suture and scarring with associated surgical trauma of the superficial palmar branch of the ulnar nerve.

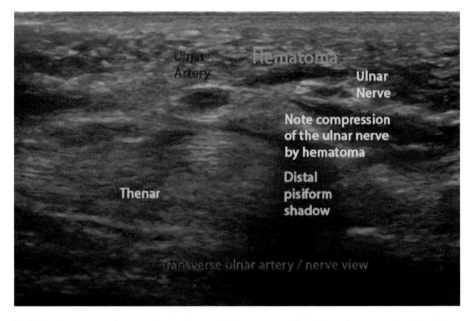

Fig. 3.15 Transverse ultrasound image demonstrating compression of the ulnar nerve by a hematoma in a patient who hammered on a hubcap with his hypothenar eminence.

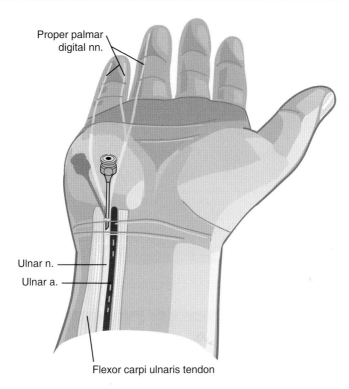

Fig. 3.16 Injection of the ulnar nerve as it passes through the ulnar tunnel with local anesthetic and/or steroid technique can serve as a diagnostic and therapeutic maneuver. (From Waldman S. *Atlas of Interventional Pain Management*. 5th ed. Philadelphia: Elsevier; 2021 [Fig. 62-7].)

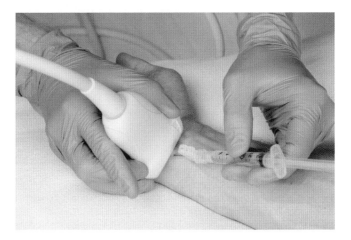

Fig. 3.17 Ultrasound-guided injection of the ulnar nerve at the ulnar canal. (From Waldman S. *Atlas of Interventional Pain Management*. 5th ed. Philadelphia: Elsevier; 2021 [Fig. 62-8].)

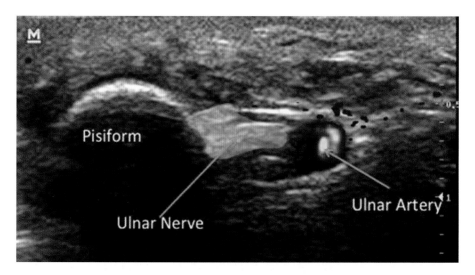

Fig. 3.18 Color Doppler can help identify the ulnar artery, which is adjacent to the ulnar nerve.

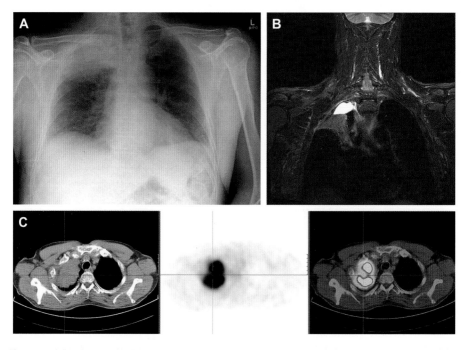

Fig. 3.19 (A) Preoperative chest x-ray demonstrates a right apical lung tumor. (B) Coronal STIR magnetic resonance imaging following induction chemoradiation demonstrates right apical lung tumor in a patient with T1 nerve root involvement. (C) Axial computed tomography (CT) scan *(left)*, axial positron emission tomography (PET) scan *(center)*, coregistered CT and PET images *(right)* demonstrating right apical lung tumor. (From Davis GA, Knight SR. Pancoast tumors. *Neurosurg Clin North Am*. 2008;19 (4):545–557 [Fig. 1]. ISSN 1042-3680, https://doi.org/10.1016/j.nec.2008.07.002, http://www.sciencedirect.com/science/article/pii/S1042368008000314.)

no reflex changes, and motor and sensory changes are limited to the distal ulnar nerve.

Diabetic polyneuropathy generally manifests as symmetric sensory deficit involving the entire hand rather than limited in the distribution of the ulnar nerve. Cervical radiculopathy and ulnar nerve entrapment may coexist as the double crush syndrome. Because ulnar tunnel syndrome is commonly seen in patients with diabetes, diabetic polyneuropathy usually occurs in patients with diabetes with ulnar tunnel syndrome. Pancoast tumor invading the medial cord of the brachial plexus also may mimic an isolated ulnar nerve entrapment and should be ruled out by apical lordotic chest radiographs.

TREATMENT

Initial treatment of the pain and functional disability associated with ulnar tunnel syndrome should include a combination of nonsteroidal antiinflammatory drugs (NSAIDs) or cyclooxygenase-2 (COX-2) inhibitors and physical therapy. Local application of heat and cold also may be beneficial. The repetitive movements that incite the syndrome should be avoided. For patients who do not respond to these treatment modalities, injection of the ulnar nerve at the ulnar tunnel with a local anesthetic and steroid may be a reasonable next step (see Figs. 3.16 and 3.17). If the symptoms of ulnar tunnel syndrome persist, surgical exploration and decompression of the ulnar nerve are indicated.

COMPLICATIONS AND PITFALLS

The major complication associated with ulnar tunnel syndrome is due to delayed diagnosis and treatment of the disease. This delay can cause permanent neurologic deficits resulting from prolonged untreated entrapment of the ulnar nerve. Failure of the clinician to recognize an acute inflammatory or infectious arthritis of the wrist may result in permanent damage to the joint and chronic pain and functional disability.

Ulnar tunnel syndrome should be differentiated from cervical radiculopathy involving the C8 spinal root, which sometimes may mimic ulnar nerve compression. Cervical radiculopathy and ulnar nerve entrapment may coexist in the double crush syndrome. The double crush syndrome is seen most commonly with ulnar nerve entrapment at the wrist or carpal tunnel syndrome. Pancoast tumor invading the medial cord of the brachial plexus also may mimic isolated ulnar nerve entrapment and should be ruled out by apical lordotic chest radiographs.

HIGH-YIELD TAKEAWAYS

- The patient is afebrile, making an acute infectious etiology unlikely.
- The patient's symptomatology is thought to be the result of compression of the ulnar nerve as it passes through the ulnar tunnel.
- Physical examination and testing should be focused on the identification of the various causes of ulnar nerve entrapment at the wrist.
- The patient exhibits the neurologic and physical examination findings that are highly suggestive of ulnar nerve entrapment at the wrist.
- The patient's symptoms are unilateral suggestive of a local process rather than a systemic inflammatory process such as rheumatoid arthritis.
- Plain radiographs will provide high-yield information regarding the bony contents of the joint, but ultrasound imaging and MRI will be more useful in identifying soft tissue pathology that may be responsible for ulnar nerve compromise.
- EMG and nerve conduction velocity testing will help delineate the location and degree of nerve compromise if ulnar nerve compromise is suspected.

Suggested Readings

Eberlin KR, Marjoua Y, Jupiter JB. Compressive neuropathy of the ulnar nerve: a perspective on history and current controversies. *J Hand Surg*. 2017;42(6):464–469.

Levina Y, Lourie GM, Matthias RC. Dynamic nerve compression of Guyon canal secondary to variation of the deep branch of the ulnar artery: etiology, diagnosis, treatment, and outcome. *J Hand Surg Global Online*. 2020;2(4):256–259.

Shen L, Masih S, Patel D, et al. MR anatomy and pathology of the ulnar nerve involving the cubital tunnel and Guyon's canal. *Clin Imaging*. 2016;40(2):263–274.

Waldman SD. Ulnar nerve. In: *Pain Review*. 2nd ed. Philadelphia: W.B. Saunders; 2017:101–102.

Waldman SD. Ulnar tunnel syndrome. In: *Atlas of Uncommon Pain Syndromes*. 4th ed. Philadelphia: Elsevier; 2020:167–170.

Waldman SD. Ulnar tunnel syndrome and other disorders of the ulnar nerve at the wrist. In: *Waldman's Comprehensive Atlas of Diagnostic Ultrasound of Painful Conditions*. Philadelphia: Wolters Kluwer; 2016:386–398.

Waldman SD. Ultrasound guided injection technique for ulnar tunnel syndrome. In: *Waldman's Comprehensive Atlas of Ultrasound Guided Pain Management Injection Techniques*. Philadelphia: Wolters Kluwer; 2014:454–462.

Waldman SD. Ultrasound guided nerve ulnar block at the wrist. In: *Waldman's Comprehensive Atlas of Ultrasound Guided Pain Management Injection Techniques*. Philadelphia: Wolters Kluwer; 2014:438–446.

Warren Billiter

A 46-Year-Old Male With Severe Wrist Pain Associated With Ulnar Deviation of the Wrist

- Learn the common causes of wrist pain.
- Develop an understanding of the unique anatomy of the wrist joint.
- Develop an understanding of the musculotendinous units that surround the wrist joint.
- Develop an understanding of the causes of de Quervain tenosynovitis.
- Develop an understanding of the differential diagnosis of de Quervain tenosynovitis.
- Learn the clinical presentation of de Quervain tenosynovitis.
- Learn how to examine the wrist.
- Learn how to use physical examination to identify de Quervain tenosynovitis.
- Develop an understanding of the treatment options for de Quervain tenosynovitis.

Warren Billiter

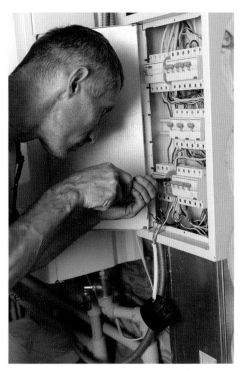

Warren Billiter is a 46-year-old electrician with the chief complaint of "I have a catch in my left wrist, and it hurts like hell." Warren stated that he just completed a huge remodel, and because they got behind, he had been putting in 14-hour days, 7 days a week for the last month. "I think that this is what caused my wrist problem. Doc, this job was brutal, but the money was good and the guy I work for was really up against it. You know how it is, one of these jobs where nothing goes right from the start."

I asked Warren about any anteent wrist trauma, and he said he had broke his arm falling out of the hay loft when he was a kid, but now it was just the usual aches and pains that go along with working with your hands. "Being an electrician ain't no spectator sport." I asked what made the pain better, and he said that a couple of Aleves washed down with a couple of Miller's seemed to help. I asked Warren what made it worse, and he said the heating pad and anything that required him using his thumb to pinch. "You know, like picking up a bolt and washer. What really kills me is picking up my new grandson. He's a real chunk. When I grab him under the arms to get him out of his crib, I almost want to whimper it hurts so bad. Twisting a screwdriver is just brutal, especially when I am tightening down something." I asked how he was sleeping, and he said, "Not worth a crap! I can't lay on my left side, and that's the side I like to sleep on." He denied fever and chills. I asked Warren to point with one finger to show me where it hurt the most. He pointed to the radial side of his left wrist. "Any other symptoms other than the pain?" I asked. "You know, Doc, I feel like the inside of my wrist is always hot and swollen. By the end of the day, it actually creaks when I move it. I'm not kidding, I can actually feel it creak, and sometimes it catches. What the hell, Doc?"

On physical examination, Warren was afebrile. His respirations were 16 and his pulse was 72 and regular. He was normotensive with a blood pressure of 120/70. Warren's head, eyes, ears, nose, throat (HEENT) exam was normal except for a big scar through his upper lip. "What happened here?" I asked as I

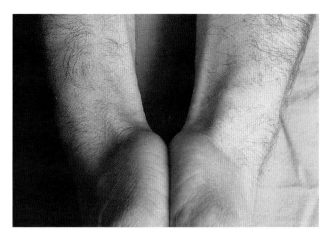

Fig. 4.1   Example of de Quervain tenosynotis of the left wrist. Note the thickening of the tendon. (From Klippel JH, Dieppe PA. *Rheumatology*, 2nd ed. Mosby: St. Louis, 1997.)

pointed to his lip. "They tell you not to walk behind a horse for a reason, Doc." I laughed and said that I would try to remember that.

His cardiopulmonary examination was completely normal. His thyroid was normal, as was his abdominal examination, which revealed no abnormal mass or organomegaly. There was no costovertebral angle (CVA) tenderness or peripheral edema. Warren's low back examination was unremarkable. Visual inspection of the left wrist revealed swelling over the radial aspect of the wrist as well as thickening of the tendons (Fig. 4.1). While there was no obvious infection, it was tender to palpation and warm to touch. I performed a Finklestein test on both wrists (Fig. 4.2). The right wrist was negative, with the left being markedly positive. I palpated the wrist while I had Warren actively ulnar deviate his wrist, and crepitus was identified. The right wrist examination was normal, as was examination of his other major joints. A careful neurologic examination of the upper extremities revealed no evidence of peripheral or entrapment neuropathy, and the deep tendon reflexes were normal.

Key Clinical Points—What's Important and What's Not

THE HISTORY

- A history of overuse of the wrist
- No history of previous significant wrist pain
- No fever or chills
- Onset of wrist pain following overuse with exacerbation of pain with wrist use

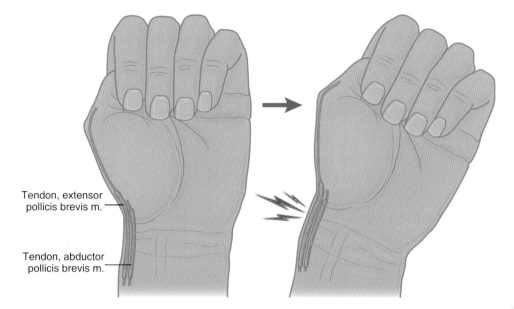

Tendon, extensor
pollicis brevis m.

Tendon, abductor
pollicis brevis m.

Fig. 4.2 A positive Finkelstein test is indicative of de Quervain tenosynovitis. (From Waldman SD. *Atlas of pain management injection techniques*. Philadelphia: Saunders; 2000.)

- Pain in the left wrist
- A catching sensation and crepitus with ulnar deviation of the left wrist
- Sleep disturbance
- Difficulty elevating and externally rotating the affected upper extremity

THE PHYSICAL EXAMINATION

- Patient is afebrile
- Tenderness to palpation of the radial aspect of the wrist
- Positive Finklestein test on the left (see Fig. 4.2)
- Palpation of radial aspect of the left wrist reveals warmth to touch
- No evidence of infection
- Crepitus with ulnar deviation of the left wrist
- Pain on range of motion, especially ulnar deviation of the wrist

OTHER FINDINGS OF NOTE

- Normal HEENT examination
- Normal cardiovascular examination
- Normal pulmonary examination
- Normal abdominal examination

- No peripheral edema
- Normal upper extremity neurologic examination, motor and sensory examination
- Examination of joints other than the left wrist was normal

 ## What Tests Would You Like to Order?

The following tests were ordered:
- Plain radiographs of the left wrist
- Ultrasound of the left radial wrist

TEST RESULTS

The plain radiographs of the left wrist reveal osteopenia of the radial wrist with associated mild soft tissue swelling (Fig. 4.3).

 ## Clinical Correlation—Putting It All Together

What is the diagnosis?
- De Quervain tenosynovitis

The Science Behind the Diagnosis

ANATOMY

De Quervain tenosynovitis is caused by inflammation and swelling of the tendons of the abductor pollicis longus and extensor pollicis brevis tendons at the level of the radial styloid process as they pass through the first dorsal compartment (Figs. 4.4 and 4.5). The abductor pollicis longus tendon is larger than the extensor pollicis brevis tendon, and these tendons may be separated by a septum in some patients (Fig. 4.6). The angle at which the abductor pollicis longus and extensor pollicis brevis tendons pass beneath the retinaculum contributes to the propensity of these tendons to become inflamed (Fig. 4.7).

CLINICAL SYNDROME

De Quervain tenosynovitis is caused by inflammation and swelling of the tendons of the abductor pollicis longus and extensor pollicis brevis tendons at the level of the radial styloid process (Fig. 4.8). This painful condition occurs most commonly between the ages of 30 and 50. It occurs more frequently in women. It is usually the result of trauma to the tendon from repetitive twisting motions. This condition is often associated with inflammatory arthritis, including rheumatoid arthritis. There

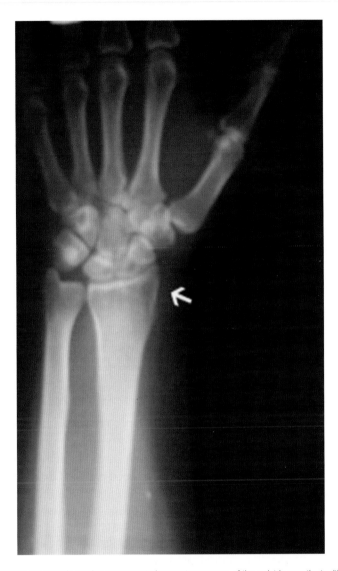

Fig. 4.3 Localized osteopenia on the anteroposterior roentgenogram of the wrist in a patient with de Quervain tenosynovitis *(arrow)*. Note mild soft tissue swelling over the radial aspect of the wrist. (From Altay MA, Erturk C, Isikan UE. De Quervain's disease treatment using partial resection of the extensor retinaculum: a short-term results survey. *Orthop Traumatol Surg Res.* 2011;97(5):489–493 [Fig. 1]. ISSN 1877-0568, https://doi.org/ 10.1016/j.otsr.2011.03.015, http://www.sciencedirect.com/science/article/pii/S187705681100106X.)

is also an association with pregnancy and baby care as lifting an infant requires using the thumbs for leverage. If the inflammation and swelling become chronic, the tendon sheath thickens, resulting in its constriction. A triggering phenomenon may occur, with the tendon catching within the sheath and causing the thumb to

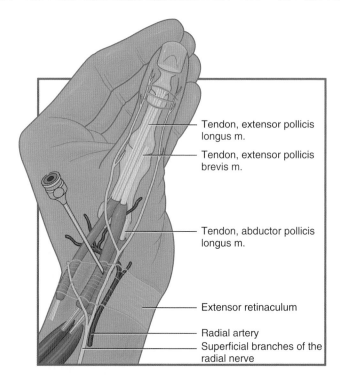

Tendon, extensor pollicis longus m.

Tendon, extensor pollicis brevis m.

Tendon, abductor pollicis longus m.

Extensor retinaculum

Radial artery

Superficial branches of the radial nerve

Fig. 4.4   Anatomy of the first dorsal compartment and injection technique for de Quervain tenosynovitis. (From Waldman S. *Atlas of Pain Management Injection Techniques*. 4th ed. St. Louis: Elsevier; 2017 [Fig. 77-2].)

lock, or "trigger." Arthritis and gout of the first metacarpal joint may coexist with de Quervain tenosynovitis and exacerbate the associated pain and disability.

De Quervain tenosynovitis occurs in patients engaged in repetitive activities such as handshaking or high-torque wrist turning (e.g., when scooping ice cream). It is also seen in new parents from repeatedly grasping their newborns between their thumbs and fingers when they pick them up. De Quervain tenosynovitis may also develop without obvious antecedent trauma.

The pain of de Quervain tenosynovitis is localized to the region of the radial styloid. It is constant and is made worse with active pinching activities of the thumb or ulnar deviation of the wrist (see Fig. 4.8). Patients note an inability to hold a coffee cup or turn a screwdriver. Sleep disturbance is common.

SIGNS AND SYMPTOMS

On physical examination, the patient has tenderness and swelling over the tendons and tendon sheaths along the distal radius, with point tenderness over the radial styloid. Many patients with de Quervain tenosynovitis note a creaking

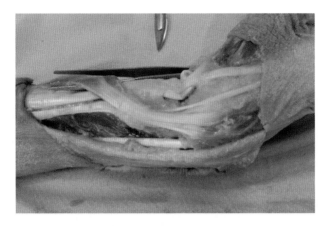

Fig. 4.5   The anatomy of the abductor pollicis longus and extensor pollicis brevis tendons at the level of the radial styloid process as they pass through the retinaculum. (From Gerlac D. De Quervain's tenosynovitis: pulling down the radius has the effect of decreasing the pain. Analysis of 36 cases. *Kinésithérapie Revue.* 2019;19(208):3−11 [Fig. 1]. ISSN 1779-0123, https://doi.org/10.1016/j.kine.2018.12.013, http://www.sciencedirect.com/science/article/pii/S1779012318304327.)

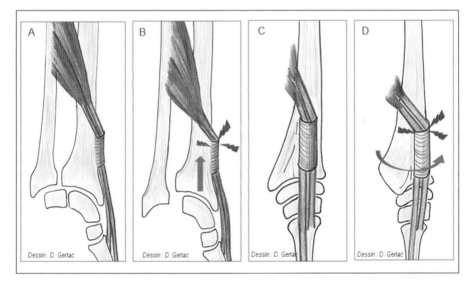

Fig. 4.6   Schematic representation of the angle of incidence of the abductor pollicis longus and extensor pollicis brevis tendons as they pass through the retinaculum and the effect of various wrist motions. (A) Wrist in neutral position. (B) Traction on Radius. (C) Radial View of Wrist in Neutral position. (D) Rotation of the radius. (From Gerlac D. De Quervain's tenosynovitis: pulling down the radius has the effect of decreasing the pain. Analysis of 36 cases. *Kinésithérapie Revue.* 2019;19(208):3−11 [Fig. 2]. ISSN 1779-0123, https://doi.org/10.1016/j.kine.2018.12.013, http://www.sciencedirect.com/science/article/pii/S1779012318304327.)

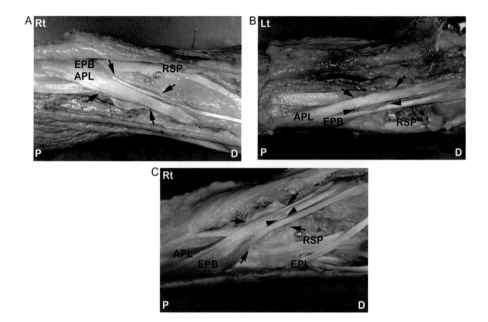

Fig. 4.7 Anatomy of de Quervain tenosysnovitis. Fibrous septum dividing the abductor pollicis longus and extensor pollicis brevis tendons within the first dorsal extensor compartment (first EC). (A) No septum, (B) complete septum, and (C) incomplete septum. This comprised 33.3% of the total length of the first dorsal extensor compartment distally. Arrows indicate the proximal and distal margins of the first dorsal extensor compartment. Arrowheads indicate the septum separating the APL and EPB. *APL*, Abductor pollicis longus; *D*, distal; *EPB*, extensor pollicis brevis; *Lt*, left; *P*, proximal; *RSP*, radial styloid process; *Rt*, right. (From Nam YS, Doh GH, Hong KY, et al. Anatomical study of the first dorsal extensor compartment for the treatment of de Quervain's disease. *Ann Anat Anatomischer Anzeiger*. 2018;218:250–255 [Fig. 1]. ISSN 0940-9602, https://doi.org/10.1016/j.aanat.2018.04.007, http://www.sciencedirect.com/science/article/pii/S0940960218300669.)

sensation with flexion and extension of the thumb. A catching or stop-and-go sensation may be present when moving the thumb. Range of motion of the thumb may be decreased by the pain, and a trigger thumb phenomenon may be noted. Patients with de Quervain tenosynovitis demonstrate a positive Finkelstein test result (see Fig. 4.2). The Finkelstein test is performed by stabilizing the patient's forearm, having the patient fully flex the thumb into the palm, and then actively forcing the wrist toward the ulna. Sudden, severe pain is highly suggestive of de Quervain tenosynovitis. Other provocative tests for de Quervain tenosynovitis include the Eickoff and Brunelli tests.

TESTING

The diagnosis is generally made on clinical grounds, but magnetic resonance imaging (MRI) and ultrasound imaging can confirm the presence of

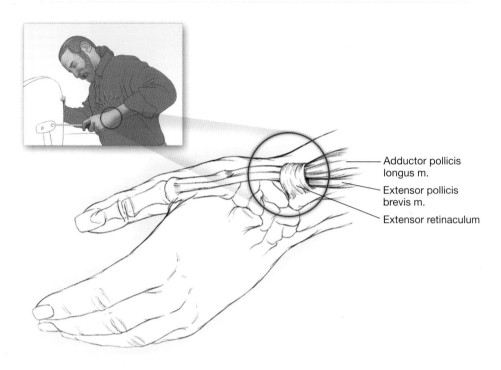

Adductor pollicis
longus m.

Extensor pollicis
brevis m.

Extensor retinaculum

Fig. 4.8   Repetitive microtrauma to the wrist can result in de Quervain tenosynovitis. (From Waldman S. *Atlas of Common Pain Syndromes*. 4th ed. Philadelphia: Elsevier; 2019 [Fig. 52-1].)

tenosynovitis (Figs. 4.9 and 4.10). Electromyography can distinguish de Quervain tenosynovitis from neuropathic processes such as cervical radiculopathy and cheiralgia paresthetica. Plain radiographs are indicated in all patients who present with de Quervain tenosynovitis to rule out occult bony disease (Fig. 4.11). Computed tomography (CT) scanning may also help further delineate the pathology thought to be responsible for the patient's pain symptomatology (Fig. 4.12). Based on the patient's clinical presentation, additional testing may be warranted, including a complete blood count, uric acid level, erythrocyte sedimentation rate, and antinuclear antibody testing. MRI and ultrasound imaging of the wrist are also indicated if joint instability is suspected and to clarify the clinical pathology responsible for the patient's symptoms (Fig. 4.13). Ultrasound evaluation will also help determine if the abductor pollicis longus and extensor pollicis tendons are separated by a septum, necessitating repositioning of the needle to determine accurate placement of corticosteroid and local anesthetic (see Fig. 4.7). The injection technique described later serves as both a diagnostic and a therapeutic maneuver.

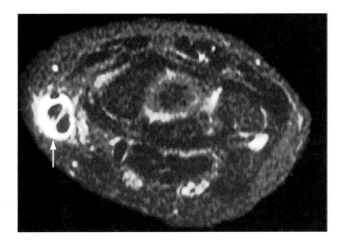

Fig. 4.9 Axial short tau inversion recovery magnetic resonance image demonstrating de Quervain tenosynovitis. Note the thickened first extensor compartment tendons, with prominent tendon sheath fluid *(arrow)*. (From Edelman RR, Hesselink JR, Zlatkin MB, Crues JV, eds. *Clinical magnetic resonance imaging*. 3rd ed. Philadelphia: Saunders; 2006:3357.)

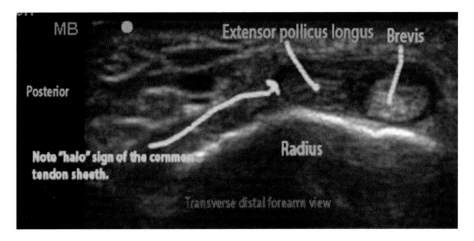

Fig. 4.10 Ultrasound image demonstrating findings consistent with de Quervain tenosynovitis. Note the halo sign indicating fluid around the tendon.

DIFFERENTIAL DIAGNOSIS

Entrapment of the lateral antebrachial cutaneous nerve, arthritis of the first metacarpal joint, gout, cheiralgia paresthetica (caused by entrapment of the superficial branch of the radial nerve at the wrist), and occasionally C6-C7

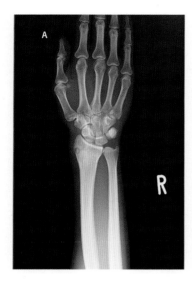
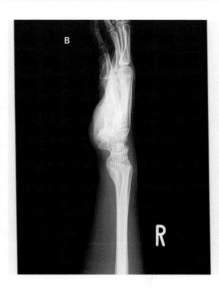

Fig. 4.11 X-ray of the right wrist with a nidus and central mineralization in a patient with a clinical diagnosis of de Quervain tenosynovitis. (A) Frontal view. (B) Lateral view. (From Iwatsuki K, Yoneda H, Kurimoto S, et al. Osteoid osteoma of the wrist misdiagnosed as de Quervain's tenosynovitis due to normal x-ray at the first visit: a case report. *Int J Surg Case Rep.* 2020;75:469—472 [Fig. 2]. ISSN 2210-2612, https://doi.org/10.1016/j.ijscr.2020.09.138, http://www.sciencedirect.com/science/article/pii/S2210261220308117.)

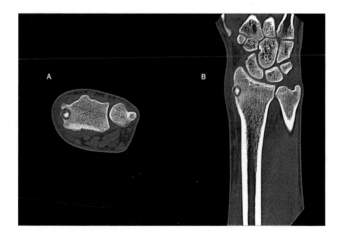

Fig. 4.12 A patient with osteoid osteoma with a clinical presentation of de Quervain tenosynovitis. Computed tomography of the right wrist with a nidus and central mineralization. (A) Axial view. (B) Coronal view. (From Iwatsuki K, Yoneda H, Kurimoto S, et al. Osteoid osteoma of the wrist misdiagnosed as de Quervain's tenosynovitis due to normal x-ray at the first visit: a case report. *Int J Surg Case Rep.* 2020;75:469—472 [Fig. 3]. ISSN 2210-2612, https://doi.org/10.1016/j.ijscr.2020.09.138, http://www.sciencedirect.com/science/article/pii/S2210261220308117.)

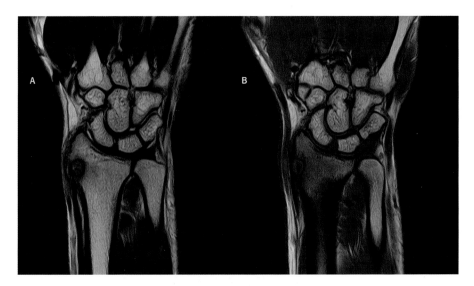

Fig. 4.13 Magnetic resonance imaging of the right wrist demonstrating an osteoid osteoma in a patient with the clinical presentation of de Quervain tenosynoviti. (A) The T2-weighted coronal view. (B) The T1-weighted coronal view. (From Iwatsuki K, Yoneda H, Kurimoto S, et al. Osteoid osteoma of the wrist misdiagnosed as de Quervain's tenosynovitis due to normal x-ray at the first visit: a case report. *Int J Surg Case Rep.* 2020;75:469—472 [Fig. 4]. ISSN 2210-2612, https://doi.org/10.1016/j.ijscr.2020.09.138, http://www.sciencedirect.com/science/article/pii/S2210261220308117.)

radiculopathy can mimic de Quervain tenosynovitis. All these painful conditions can also coexist with de Quervain tenosynovitis (Table 4.1).

TREATMENT

Initial treatment of the pain and functional disability associated with de Quervain tenosynovitis includes a combination of nonsteroidal antiinflammatory drugs (NSAIDs) or cyclooxygenase-2 inhibitors and physical therapy. Local application of heat and cold may also be beneficial. Any repetitive activity that may exacerbate the patient's symptoms should be avoided. Nighttime splinting of the affected thumb may help avoid the trigger phenomenon that can occur on awakening in many patients suffering from this condition. For patients who do not respond to these treatment modalities, injection of the first dorsal compartment of the wrist with local anesthetic and/or steroid is a reasonable next step. Ultrasound guidance will increase the accuracy of needle placement and decrease the incidence of needle-induced complications (Fig. 4.14). The injection of platelet-rich plasma and/or stem cells around the inflamed tendons may aid in the resolution of symptoms associated with de Quervain tenosynovitis.

TABLE 4.1 ■ **Differential Diagnosis of de Quervain Tenosynovitis**

- Abnormalities of the radial styloid
- Fractures of the scaphoid
- Intersection syndrome
- C6 radiculopathy
- Keinboch disease
- Arthritis of the carpophalangeal joint of the thumb
- Cheiragia paresthetica (wristwatch palsy)
- Tumor
- Infection
- Ganglion cysts
- Entrapment neuropathies of the wrist
- Synostosis of the scaphoid and trapezium

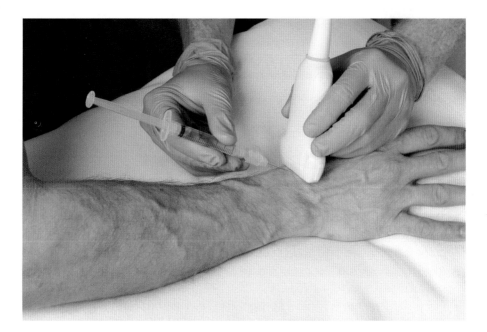

Fig. 4.14   Ultrasound injection of de Quervain tenosynovitis.

Ultrasound-guided needle placement will aid in the accurate needle placement in patients suffering from de Quervain tenosynovitis. Physical modalities, including local heat and gentle range-of-motion exercises, should be introduced several days after the patient undergoes injection. Splinting may provide symptomatic relief. Vigorous exercises should be avoided because they will exacerbate the patient's symptoms.

COMPLICATIONS AND PITFALLS

The injection technique is safe if careful attention is paid to the clinically relevant anatomy. The radial artery and superficial branch of the radial nerve are susceptible to damage if the needle is placed too medially, so care must be taken to avoid these structures. The major complications associated with injection are related to trauma to the inflamed and previously damaged tendons. These tendons may rupture if they are injected directly, so the needle position should be confirmed to be outside the tendon before injection. Another complication of injection is infection, although it should be exceedingly rare if strict aseptic technique is followed, as well as universal precautions to minimize any risk to the operator. The incidence of ecchymosis and hematoma formation can be decreased if pressure is applied to the injection site immediately after injection. Approximately 25% of patients complain of a transient increase in pain after injection, and patients should be warned of this possibility.

HIGH-YIELD TAKEAWAYS

- The patient is afebrile, making an acute infectious etiology (e.g., septic arthritis) unlikely.
- The patient's symptomatology is the result of overuse of the wrist, and physical examination and testing should be focused on the identification of ligamentous injury, tendinitis, acute arthritis, and bursitis.
- The patient has point tenderness over the radial aspect of the wrist, which is highly suggestive of de Quervain tenosynovitis.
- There is warmth over the affected joint suggestive of an inflammatory process.
- The patient's symptoms are unilateral, which is more suggestive of a local process than a systemic polyarthropathy or collagen vascular disease.
- Sleep disturbance is common and must be addressed concurrently with the patient's pain symptomatology.
- Plain radiographs will provide high-yield information regarding the bony contents of the joint, but ultrasound imaging and MRI will be more useful in identifying soft tissue pathology. CT imaging may also help clarify the etiology of bony abnormalities identified on x-ray.

Suggested Readings

O'Neill CJ. de Quervain tenosynovitis. In: Frontera WR, Silver JK, Rizzo TD, eds. *Essentials of Physical Medicine and Rehabilitation*. 4th ed. Philadelphia: Elsevier; 2020:149–153.

Waldman SD. de Quervain's tenosynovitis. In: *Pain Review*. 2nd ed. Philadelphia: Elsevier; 2017:261–263.

Waldman SD. De Quervain tenosynovitis. In: *Waldman's Comprehensive Atlas of Diagnostic Ultrasound of Painful Conditions*. Philadelphia: Wolters Kluwer; 2016:417–424.

Waldman SD. Functional anatomy of the wrist. In: *Pain Review*. 2nd ed. Philadelphia: Elsevier; 2017:106.

Waldman SD. Injection technique for de Quervain tenosynovitis. In: *Atlas of Pain Management Injection Techniques*. 4th ed. Philadelphia: Saunders; 2017:278–281.

Waldman SD. Intra-articular injection of the wrist joint. In: *Atlas of Pain Management Injection Techniques*. 4th ed. Philadelphia: Elsevier; 2017:250–253.

Waldman SD. Painful conditions of the wrist and hand. In: *Physical Diagnosis of Pain: An Atlas of Signs and Symptoms*. 4th ed. Philadelphia: Elsevier; 2021:184.

Waldman SD. The Finkelstein test for de Quervain tenosynovitis. In: *Physical Diagnosis of Pain: An Atlas of Signs and Symptoms*. 4th ed. Philadelphia: Elsevier; 2021:187–189.

Stefon Dawson

A 26-Year-Old Male With Severe Dorsal Wrist Pain Associated With Flexion and Extension of the Wrist

LEARNING OBJECTIVES

- Learn the common causes of wrist pain.
- Develop an understanding of the unique anatomy of the wrist joint.
- Develop an understanding of the musculotendinous units that surround the wrist joint.
- Develop an understanding of the causes of intersection syndrome.
- Develop an understanding of the differential diagnosis of intersection syndrome.
- Learn how to distinguish intersection syndrome from de Quervain tenosynovitis.
- Learn the clinical presentation of intersection syndrome.
- Learn how to examine the wrist.
- Learn how to use physical examination to identify intersection syndrome.
- Develop an understanding of the treatment options for intersection syndrome.

Stefon Dawson

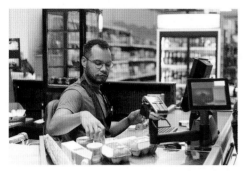

Stefon Dawson is a 26-year-old cashier at the local grocery with the chief complaint of "every time I bend my wrist, it really hurts." Stefon went on to say that the grocery store had been really short-staffed so he had been working a lot of overtime, and it was taking its toll. "I bet I pick up 10,000 groceries a day! And when Coke or Pepsi is on sale, I know its going to be really rough. I tell the customers to leave the soda pop in their cart, but they put it on the belt anyway. It's awkward and heavy to lift. I think this and the watermelons have really done in my wrist."

I asked Stefon about any antecedent wrist trauma, and he said no, he had twisted his ankle skateboarding when he was a kid, but had no previous broken bones. I asked Stefon what made the pain better, and he said that he felt like Motrin was helping, but it ate a hole in his stomach, so now he is using an ice pack on his wrist when he gets home at night. I asked Stefon what made it worse, and he said the heating pad and anything that required him to bend his wrist up or down. "How about side to side?" I inquired. "Not so much," said Stefon. "It's when I bend it up or down. You know—flex and unflex it—that it hurts. When I'm trying to get the scanner to read a code on a carton of ice cream with ice crystals, there is a lot of up and down." I asked, "What about picking things up between your thumb and index finger?" Stefan reported, "Not so much." I asked how he was sleeping, and he said, "Not very good. Whenever I bend my wrist, I get a sharp pain that wakes me up." I asked, "Does the pain go down into your fingers?" He responded, "Not really, it's pretty much on the top of my wrist over toward the right." Stefon denied fever and chills. I asked Stefon to point with one finger to show me where it hurt the most. He pointed to the radial side of the dorsum of his right wrist. "Any other symptoms other than the pain?" I asked. "You know, Doc. I feel like the top of my wrist is always hot and swollen, and by the end of the day it actually creaks when I move it up and down. This is really painful. Do you think I broke something lifting all those big watermelons?"

On physical examination, Stefon was afebrile. His respirations were 16, and his pulse was 72 and regular. He was normotensive with a blood pressure of 120/70. Stefon's head, eyes, ears, nose, throat (HEENT) exam was completely normal. His cardiopulmonary examination was completely normal. His thyroid was normal as was his abdominal examination, which revealed no abnormal mass or organomegaly. There was no costovertebral (CVA) tenderness or

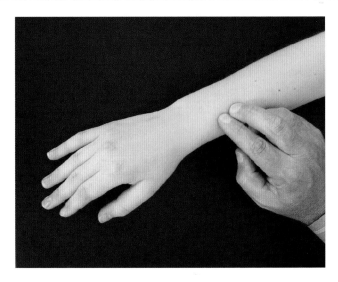

Fig. 5.1   The creaking tendon test for intersection syndrome. (From Waldman S. *Physical Diagnosis of Pain: An Atlas of Signs and Symptoms*. 4th ed. Philadelphia: Elsevier; 2021 [Fig. 105-2]. 9780323712606.)

peripheral edema. Stefon's low back examination was unremarkable. Visual inspection of the right wrist revealed swelling over the radial aspect of the dorsum of the wrist. While there was no obvious infection, it was tender to palpation and warm to touch. Stefon had a positive creaking tendon test on the right (Fig. 5.1). The left wrist creaking tendon was negative. I palpated the wrist while I had Stefon actively ulnar flex and extend his wrist against resistance, which recreated his pain. Crepitus was identified. There was only minimal pain with ulnar deviation of the right wrist. The left wrist examination was normal, as was examination of his other major joints. A careful neurologic examination of the upper extremities revealed no evidence of peripheral or entrapment neuropathy, and the deep tendon reflexes were normal.

Key Clinical Points—What's Important and What's Not

THE HISTORY

- A history of overuse of the wrist
- No history of previous significant wrist pain or injury
- No fever or chills
- Pain localized to the radial side of the dorsum of the wrist

- Onset of wrist pain following overuse with exacerbation of pain with flexion and extension of the wrist
- Minimal pain with ulnar deviation of the wrist
- Pain in the right wrist
- Crepitus over the radial side of the dorsum of the right wrist with flexion and extension
- Sleep disturbance

THE PHYSICAL EXAMINATION

- Patient is afebrile
- Tenderness to palpation of the radial aspect of the dorsum of the right wrist
- Positive creaking tendon test on the right (see Fig. 5.1)
- Palpation of radial aspect of the dorsum right wrist reveals warmth to touch
- No evidence of infection
- Crepitus over the radial aspect of the dorsum right wrist with flexion and extension of the right wrist
- Pain on range of motion, especially ulnar deviation of the wrist

OTHER FINDINGS OF NOTE

- Normal HEENT examination
- Normal cardiovascular examination
- Normal pulmonary examination
- Normal abdominal examination
- No peripheral edema
- Normal upper extremity neurologic examination, motor and sensory examination
- Examination of joints other than the right wrist is normal

 What Tests Would You Like to Order?

The following tests were ordered:
- Ultrasound of the right wrist
- Magnetic resonance imaging (MRI) of the right wrist

TEST RESULTS

The ultrasound imaging of the right wrist demonstrated fluid surrounding the intersection of the first extensor compartment (abductor pollicis longus tendon) and the

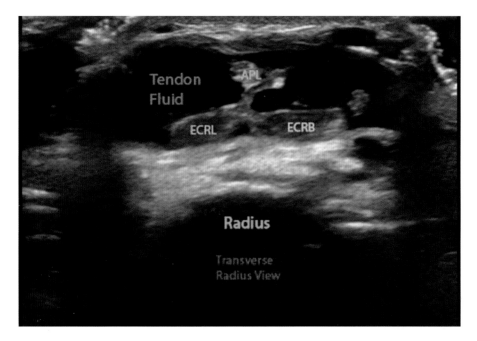

Fig. 5.2   Transverse ultrasound image of intersection syndrome. Note the significant fluid accumulation around the tendons.

second extensor compartment (extensor carpi radialis longus and extensor carpi radialis), which is consistent with a diagnosis of intersection syndrome (Fig. 5.2).

Clinical Correlation—Putting It All Together

What is the diagnosis?
- Intersection syndrome

The Science Behind the Diagnosis
ANATOMY

Intersection syndrome involves the first two compartments of the six compartments that house the extensor tendons of the distal dorsal forearm and dorsal wrist. Passing obliquely over the extensor carpi radialis brevis and extensor carpi radialis longus tendons of the second compartment, the abductor pollicis longus and extensor pollicis brevis of the first compartment intersect at their musculotendinous junctions (Fig. 5.3). This intersection is just proximal to the extensor retinaculum, which serves to tether down the tendons and may contribute to the evolution of intersection syndrome (Fig. 5.4).

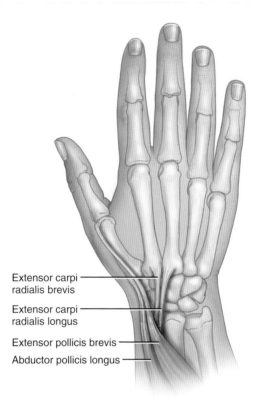

Extensor carpi
radialis brevis

Extensor carpi
radialis longus

Extensor pollicis brevis

Abductor pollicis longus

Fig. 5.3   Intersection syndrome. Site of the intersection of the tendons responsible for the clinical syndrome. (From Waldman S. *Atlas of Pain Management Injection Techniques*. 4th ed. St. Louis: Elsevier; 2017 [Fig. 78-1].)

CLINICAL SYNDROME

Intersection syndrome gets its name because it is caused by tenosynovitis at the inter-section of the first and second extensor compartments (see Figs. 5.3 and 5.4). Intersection syndrome is also known as ice axe and oarsman's wrist among a variety of other names because of the increased incidence of this painful condition in climbers and rowers (Table 5.1). The tendons within these compartments that become inflamed include the extensor carpi radialis longus, the extensor carpi radialis brevis, the extensor pollicis brevis, and the abductor pollicis longus tendons and associated muscles (Fig. 5.5). This inflammation can be a result of direct trauma to the musculotendinous units or a result of overuse or misuse during activities that require repetitive flexion and extension of the wrist. Rowers, scullers, grocery cashiers, and weightlifters are at risk for developing intersection syndrome because of the repetitive flexion and exten-sion of the wrist required for these activities. Intersection syndrome is also seen with increased incidence in racquet sports, baseball, cycling, hockey, golf, ice hockey, mountain climbing, skiing, and softball (Fig. 5.6).

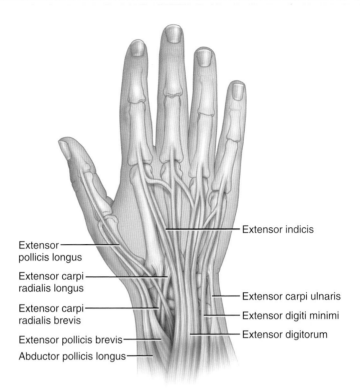

Extensor indicis

Extensor
pollicis longus

Extensor carpi
radialis longus

Extensor carpi ulnaris

Extensor carpi
radialis brevis

Extensor digiti minimi

Extensor pollicis brevis

Extensor digitorum

Abductor pollicis longus

Fig. 5.4   The relationship of the extensor retinaculum to the tendons involved in intersection syndrome. (From Waldman S. *Atlas of Pain Management Injection Techniques*. 4th ed. St. Louis: Elsevier; 2017 [Fig. 78-5].)

TABLE 5.1 ▤ Intersection Syndrome—Various Names

- Intersection syndrome
- Oarsman's wrist
- Bugaboo wrist
- Ice axe wrist
- Mountain climber's wrist
- Peritendinitis crepitans
- Crossover syndrome
- Squeaker's wrist
- Grocery store wrist

SIGNS AND SYMPTOMS

Patients with intersection syndrome will complain bitterly of radial-sided dorsal wrist pain made worse with wrist flexion or extension. The examiner may be

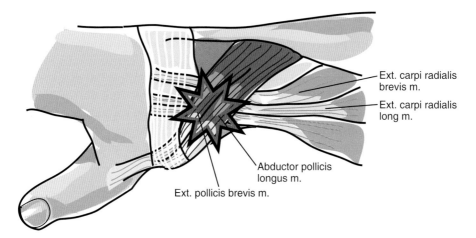

Ext. carpi radialis brevis m.

Ext. carpi radialis long m.

Abductor pollicis longus m.

Ext. pollicis brevis m.

Fig. 5.5 Intersection syndrome. Relevant soft tissue anatomy. (From Waldman S. *Physical Diagnosis of Pain: An Atlas of Signs and Symptoms*. 4th ed. Philadelphia: Elsevier; 2021 [Fig. 105-1].)

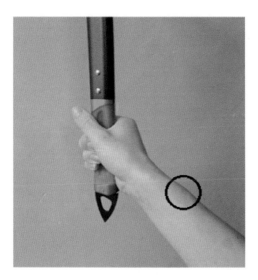

Fig. 5.6 Intersection syndrome. Site of pain. Image of ice axe in hand with area of intersection highlighted. (From "Ice axe wrist": a case report of intersection syndrome in two climbers. *Wilderness Environ Med*. 2017;28(3):230—233 [Fig. 2]. ISSN 1080-6032, https://doi.org/10.1016/j.wem.2017.03.016, http://www.sciencedirect.com/science/article/pii/S1080603217301072.)

able to elicit a positive creaking tendon test if the tendons are acutely inflamed (see Fig. 5.2). The examiner may also be able to identify what has been described as wet leather crepitus by careful palpation of the point of intersection during passive or active range of motion of the wrist. As the disease progresses, swelling at the site of intersection is invariably present.

TESTING

On the basis of the patient's clinical presentation, additional testing, including complete blood count, sedimentation rate, and antinuclear antibody testing, may be indicated. Ultrasound imaging may also help confirm the diagnosis as well as aid in needle placement when performing this injection technique (Figs. 5.7 and 5.8). MRI of the wrist is indicated if tendon rupture is suspected and to further confirm the diagnosis. Radionuclide bone scanning is useful to identify stress fractures of the wrist not seen on plain radiographs.

DIFFERENTIAL DIAGNOSIS

Other pain syndromes that cause radial-sided wrist pain and must be ruled out when considering the diagnosis of intersection syndrome include de Quervain tenosynovitis, arthritis of the carpometacarpal joint of the thumb, tendinitis of the

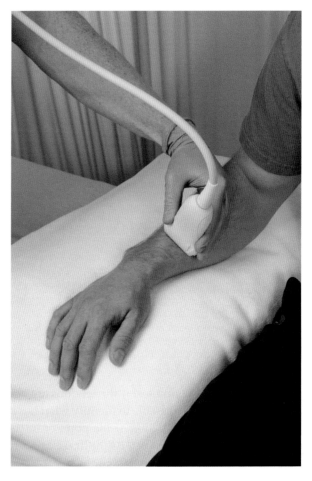

Fig. 5.7 Proper transverse position of the linear high-frequency ultrasound transducer to perform ultrasound evaluation for intersection syndrome.

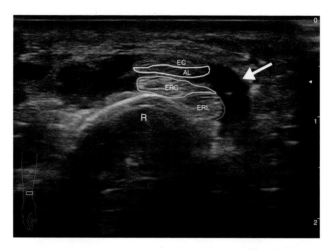

Fig. 5.8   Transverse ultrasound image of the distal region of the right forearm. Showing tenosynovitis *(arrow)* of the tendons of the I and II extensor compartment as they cross. *AL*, Abductor longus of the first finger; *EB*, extensor brevis of the first finger; *ECRB*, extensor carpi radialis brevis; *ECRL*, extensor carpi radialis longus; *R*, radius. (From Moratalla CP, Caceres BAB, Corral JB. Distal intersection syndrome: an unusual cause of forearm pain. *Reumatol Clín (English Edition)*. 2020;16(2):128—129 [Fig. 1]. ISSN 2173-5743, https://doi.org/10.1016/j.reumae.2018.02.002, http://www.sciencedirect.com/science/article/pii/S2173574319300656.)

TABLE 5.2 ■ **Differential Diagnosis of Intersection Syndrome**

- De Quervain tenosynovitis
- Abnormalities of the radial styloid
- Fractures of the scaphoid
- C6 radiculopathy
- Keinboch disease
- Arthritis of the base of the thumb
- Cheiragia paresthetica (wristwatch palsy)
- Tumor
- Infection
- Ganglion cysts
- Entrapment neuropathies of the wrist
- Synostosis of the scaphoid and trapezium

---

extensor pollicis longus, and Wartenberg syndrome (Table 5.2). Although the pain of intersection syndrome occurs more dorsally than the more radially located pain of de Quervain tenosynovitis, the two are frequently confused (Fig. 5.9). Table 5.3 compares and contrasts these two painful conditions of the radial side of the wrist.

TREATMENT

Initial treatment of the pain and functional disability associated with intersection syndrome includes a combination of nonsteroidal antiinflammatory drugs

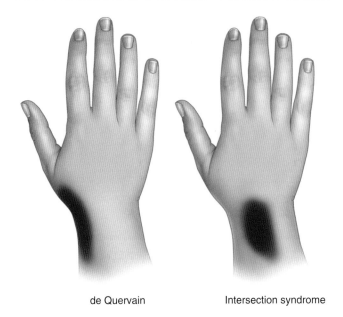

de Quervain   Intersection syndrome

Fig. 5.9   Site of pain in de Quervain tenosynovitis and intersection syndrome. (From Waldman S. *Atlas of Pain Management Injection Techniques*. 4th ed. St. Louis: Elsevier; 2017 [Fig. 78-2].)

TABLE 5.3 ■ Comparison of Intersection Syndrome With de Quervain Tenosynovitis

	Intersection Syndrome	de Quervain Tenosynovitis
Tendons involved	Extensor carpi radialis longus, extensor carpi radialis brevis, extensor pollicis brevis, abductor pollicis longus	Abductor pollicis longus, extensor pollicis brevis
Alternate names	Washerwoman's wrist	Oarsman's wrist
Clinical signs	Creaking tendon sign, wet leather crepitus	Finkelstein sign
Location of pain	7 cm above radial styloid	At the radial styloid
Site of injection	Above radial styloid at point of maximal tenderness	At the radial styloid
Frequency	Rare	Common

(NSAIDs) or cyclooxygenase-2 inhibitors and physical therapy. Local application of heat and cold may also be beneficial. Any repetitive activity that may exacerbate the patient's symptoms should be avoided. Nighttime splinting of the wrist may help avoid the nighttime pain experienced by many patients suffering from this condition. For patients who do not respond to these treatment modalities, injection of the intersection of the first and second compartments of the wrist with local anesthetic and/or steroid is a reasonable next step (Fig. 5.10).

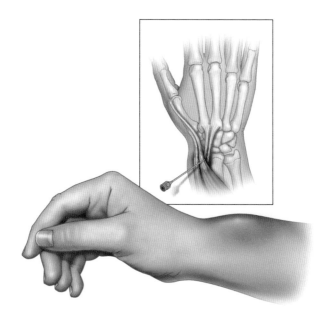

Fig. 5.10   Injection technique for intersection syndrome. (From Waldman S. *Atlas of Pain Management Injection Techniques*. 4th ed. St. Louis: Elsevier; 2017 [Fig. 78-6].)

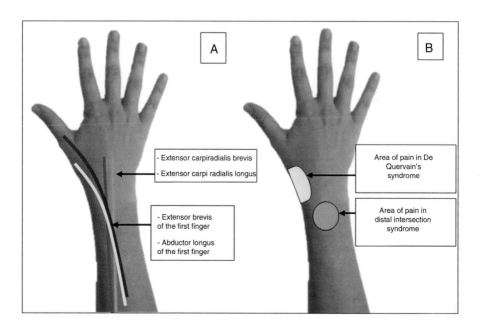

Fig. 5.11   (A) Anatomic path of the tendons involved in distal intersection syndrome. (B) Site of pain in distal intersection syndrome and in De Quervain tendonitis. (From Moratalla CP, Caceres BAB, Corral JB. Distal intersection syndrome: an unusual cause of forearm pain. *Reumatol Clín (English Edition)*. 2020;16(2, Part 1):128–129 [Fig. 2]. ISSN 2173-5743, https://doi.org/10.1016/j.reumae.2018.02.002.)

Ultrasound guidance will increase the accuracy of needle placement and decrease the incidence of needle-induced complications (Fig. 5.11). The injection of platelet-rich plasma and/or stem cells around the inflamed tendons may aid in the resolution of symptoms associated with intersection syndrome. Ultrasound-guided needle placement will aid in the accurate needle placement in patients suffering from intersection syndrome. Physical modalities, including local heat and gentle range-of-motion exercises, should be introduced several days after the patient undergoes injection. Splinting may provide symptomatic relief. Vigorous exercises should be avoided because they will exacerbate the patient's symptoms.

HIGH-YIELD TAKEAWAYS

- The patient is afebrile, making an acute infectious etiology (e.g., septic arthritis) unlikely.
- The patient's symptomatology is the result of overuse of the wrist, and physical examination and testing should be focused on the identification of ligamentous injury, tendinitis, acute arthritis, and bursitis.
- The patient has point tenderness over the radial aspect of the dorsum of the wrist, which is highly suggestive of intersection syndrome.
- There is warmth over the area, which is suggestive of an inflammatory process.
- The patient's symptoms are unilateral, which is more suggestive of a local process than a systemic polyarthropathy or connective tissue disorder.
- Sleep disturbance is common and must be addressed concurrently with the patient's pain symptomatology.
- Plain radiographs will provide high-yield information regarding the bony contents of the joint, but ultrasound imaging and MRI will be more useful in identifying soft tissue pathology. CT imaging may also help clarify the etiology of bony abnormalities identified on x-ray.

Suggested Readings

Montechiarello S, Miozzi F, D'Ambrosio I, et al. The intersection syndrome: ultrasound findings and their diagnostic value. *J Ultrasound*. 2010;13(2):70–73.

Moratalla CP, Caceres BAB, Corral JB. Distal intersection syndrome: an unusual cause of forearm pain. *Reumatol Clín (English Edition)*. 2020;16(2):128–129.

Tobin AL. "Ice axe wrist": a case report of intersection syndrome in 2 climbers. *Wilderness Environ Med*. 2017;28(3):230–233.

Waldman SD. Comprehensive atlas of ultrasound-guided pain management injection techniques. In: *Ultrasound-Guided Injection Technique for Eagle Syndrome*. New York: Wolters Kluwer; 2020:95–103.

Waldman SD. Injection technique for intersection syndrome. In: *Atlas of Pain Management Injection Techniques*. 4th ed. Elsevier; 2017:282–285.

CHAPTER

6

Victor Flores

A 36-Year-Old Male With Pain and Paresthesias Radiating Into the Base of the Thumb

LEARNING OBJECTIVES

- Learn the common causes of wrist pain and hand pain.
- Learn the common causes of hand numbness.
- Develop an understanding of the unique relationship of the superficial radial nerve to the bones of the wrist.
- Develop an understanding of the anatomy of the superficial radial nerve.
- Develop an understanding of the causes of cheiralgia paresthetica.
- Develop an understanding of the differential diagnosis of cheiralgia paresthetica.
- Learn the clinical presentation of cheiralgia paresthetica.
- Learn how to examine the wrist.
- Learn how to examine the superficial radial nerve.
- Learn how to use physical examination to identify cheiralgia paresthetica.
- Develop an understanding of the treatment options for cheiralgia paresthetica.

Victor Flores

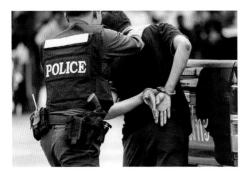

"I didn't see this one coming, Doc," said Victor. "We all have to speak up, but I didn't think that speaking up would cost me my job." Victor Flores is a 36-year-old dental lab technician with the chief complaint of "I am getting electric shocks from my wrist that shoot into the base of my thumb ever since I got handcuffed at the protest for social justice last month." Victor stated that the police sat him on the curb with the handcuffs on for about 10 hours. He said that he repeatedly complained that the handcuffs were too tight, but his complaints were ignored. He said that after a while, his right hand went numb and then just ached. Eventually, the police took off the handcuffs and told him to get out of there. "I was so glad to get those handcuffs off. It wasn't until the next day when I realized that my thumb was still numb. And I keep getting the electric shocklike jolts into the base of my thumb. It is really annoying." I asked Victor if he had experienced any other numbness or weakness, and he replied, "Doc, it's funny that you asked as I have started noticing that the back of my hand feels kind of like it's made of wood—kind of numb, with a dead feeling. It doesn't sound like a big deal, but it makes it impossible to do my work. I use my hands all day long making dentures and dental crowns. The numbness and electric shocks made it impossible for me to hold my tools, and eventually my supervisor told me that he was going to have to let me go as he was getting too many complaints about my work from our customers."

I asked Victor what he had tried to make his symptoms better, and he said that nothing he had tried had given him much relief. "My sleep is all jacked up because the electric shocks jolt me awake when I roll over." I asked Victor to describe any numbness associated with his pain, and he pointed to the radial aspect of the dorsum of his right hand, and he then rubbed the back of his thumb, index, and middle fingers. "Doc, a couple of things, or maybe I am just imagining them, but only half of my ring finger is numb, and the numbness doesn't go all the way down to the tips of the fingers. Do you think I am imagining this? It just doesn't make any sense." I asked Victor about any fever, chills, or other constitutional symptoms such as weight loss, night sweats, etc., and he shook his head no. He denied any antecedent wrist trauma or anything else that might account for his symptoms.

I asked Victor to point with one finger to show me where it hurt the most. He pointed to the base of his right thumb. He went on to say that he could live with the numbness, but the electric shocks were really bothering.

On physical examination, Victor was afebrile. His respirations were 16, his pulse was 72 and regular, and his blood pressure was 120/70. Victor's head, eyes, ears, nose, throat (HEENT) exam was normal, as was his cardiopulmonary exam. His thyroid was normal. His abdominal examination revealed no abnormal mass or organomegaly. There was no costovertebral angle (CVA) tenderness. There was no peripheral edema. His low back examination was unremarkable. Visual inspection of the right wrist was unremarkable. There was no rubor or color. There was no obvious infection or olecranon bursitis. There was a positive Tinel sign over the superficial radial nerve at the wrist (Fig. 6.1). I performed the wristwatch test, which was markedly positive on the right and equivocal on the left (Fig. 6.2). A careful neurologic examination of the upper extremities revealed decreased sensation in the distribution of the right superficial radial nerve (Fig. 6.3). "Victor, I think those handcuffs damaged a nerve in your wrist, and that is what is causing your symptoms."

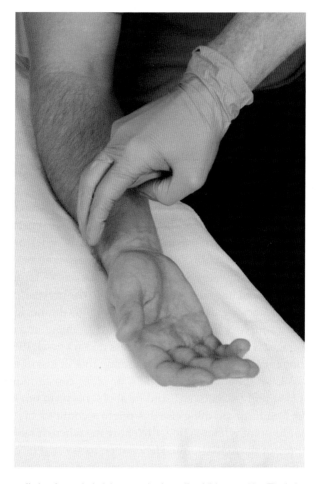

Fig. 6.1 Patients suffering from cheiralgia paresthetica will exhibit a positive Tinel sign over the superficial radial nerve.

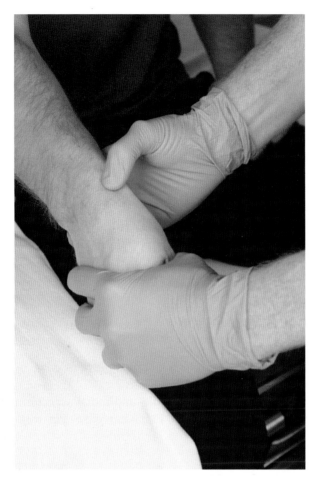

Fig. 6.2   The wristwatch test for chieralgia paresthetica is performed by having the patient fully deviate the wrist to the ulnar side. The examiner then exerts firm pressure on the skin overlying the radial nerve.

Key Clinical Points—What's Important and What's Not

THE HISTORY

- A history of the onset of symptoms after patient was placed in tight handcuffs for a 10-hour period
- A history of the onset of right hand pain with associated paresthesias and numbness radiating into the distribution of the superficial radial nerve
- Numbness of the dorsal aspect of the thumb, index, middle, and radial aspect of the ring finger with sparing of the finger tips
- No history of previous significant wrist, hand, or finger pain
- No fever or chills

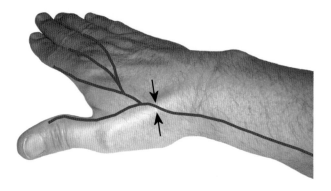

Fig. 6.3   The sensory distribution of the superficial radial nerve. (From Preston DC, Shapiro BE, eds. Radial neuropathy. In: *Electromyography and Neuromuscular Disorders*. 3rd ed. London: Saunders; 2013:331–345.)

THE PHYSICAL EXAMINATION

- Patient is afebrile
- Positive Tinel sign over the superficial radial nerve (see Fig. 6.1)
- Positive wristwatch test (see Fig. 6.2)
- Numbness of the thumb, index, middle, and radial aspect of the ring finger in the distribution of the superficial radial nerve (see Fig. 6.3)
- No evidence of infection

OTHER FINDINGS OF NOTE

- Normal HEENT examination
- Normal cardiovascular examination
- Normal pulmonary examination
- Normal abdominal examination
- No peripheral edema
- Normal left upper extremity neurologic examination, motor and sensory examination

What Tests Would You Like to Order?

The following tests were ordered:
- Ultrasound of the right wrist
- Electromyography (EMG) and nerve conduction velocity testing of the right upper extremity

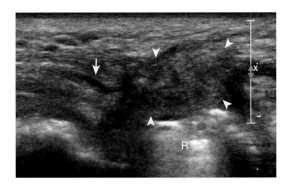

Fig. 6.4 Radial nerve, superficial branch: scar tissue. Ultrasound image shows the superficial branch of the radial nerve in long axis *(arrow)* entering into hypoechoic scar tissue and hematoma *(arrowheads)* after surgical repair of distal radius *(R)* fracture. (From Jacobson J. *Fundamentals of Musculoskeletal Ultrasound*. 3rd ed. Philadelphia: Saunders; 2018 [Fig. 5-74].)

TEST RESULTS

Ultrasound examination of the right wrist revealed superficial branch of the radial nerve surrounded by scar tissue and hematoma (Fig. 6.4).

EMG and nerve conduction velocity testing revealed slowing of superficial radial nerve conduction across the wrist as well as denervation of the intrinsic muscles of the hand.

 Clinical Correlation—Putting It All Together

What is the diagnosis?
- Cheiralgia paresthetica

The Science Behind the Diagnosis

ANATOMY

Arising from fibers from the C5-T1 nerve roots of the posterior cord of the brachial plexus, the radial nerve passes through the axilla lying posterior and inferior to the axillary artery. As the radial nerve exits the axilla, it passes between the medial and long heads of the triceps muscle and then curves across the posterior aspect of the humerus, giving off a motor branch to the triceps muscle (Fig. 6.5). Continuing its downward path, the radial nerve gives off a number of sensory branches to the upper arm as it travels in the intermuscular septum separating the bellies of the brachialis and brachioradialis muscles. The nerve passes into the substance of the brachioradialis muscle and at a point just above the lateral epicondyle, the radial nerve divides into deep and superficial branches

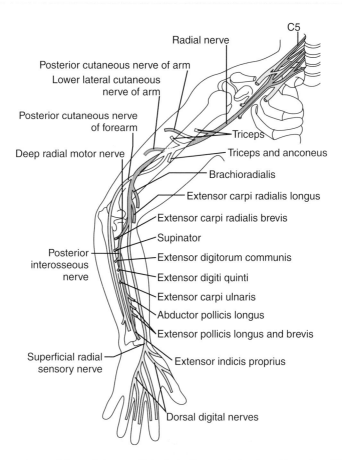

Fig. 6.5   The anatomy of the radial nerve. (Adapted with permission from Haymaker, W., Woodhall, B., 1953. *Peripheral Nerve Injuries*. WB Saunders, Philadelphia.)

(Fig. 6.6). The superficial branch of the radial nerve continues down the arm along with the radial artery to provide sensory innervation to the dorsum of the wrist and the dorsal aspects of a portion of the thumb and index and middle fingers (Figs. 6.7 and 6.8). The deep branch of the radial nerve provides the majority of the motor innervation to the extensors of the forearm.

CLINICAL SYNDROME

Cheiralgia paresthetica is an uncommon cause of wrist and hand pain and numbness. It also is known as handcuff neuropathy, prisoner's palsy, and Wartenberg syndrome. The onset of symptoms usually occurs after compression of the sensory branch of the radial nerve. Radial nerve dysfunction secondary to compression by tight handcuffs, wristwatch bands, tumor, neuroma, or casts is a common cause of cheiralgia paresthetica (Figs. 6.9 and 6.10). Direct trauma to

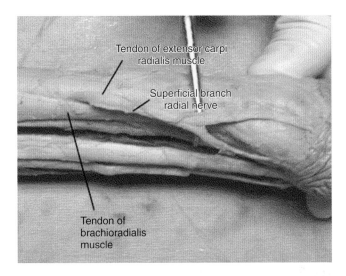

Fig. 6.6 The radial nerve passes into the substance of the brachioradialis muscle; at a point just above the lateral epicondyle, the radial nerve divides into deep and superficial branches. (From Pratt N. Anatomy of nerve entrapment sites in the upper quarter. *J Hand Ther.* 2005;18(2):216–229.)

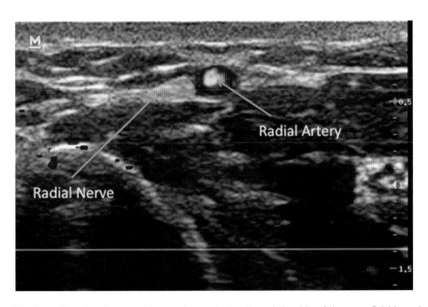

Fig. 6.7 Color Doppler ultrasound image demonstrating the relationship of the superficial branch of the radial nerve to the radial artery.

the nerve may result in a similar clinical presentation. Fractures or lacerations frequently disrupt the nerve completely, resulting in sensory deficit in the distribution of the radial nerve. The sensory branch of the radial nerve also may be damaged during surgical treatment of de Quervain tenosynovitis.

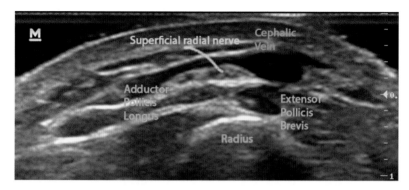

Fig. 6.8   The normal superficial radial nerve will appear as a bundle of hyperechoic nerve fibers surrounded by a slightly more hyperechoic neural sheath lying adjacent to the radial artery.

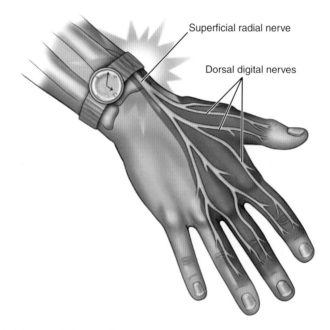

Fig. 6.9   Cheiralgia paresthetica manifests as pain, paresthesias, and numbness of the radial aspect
of the dorsum of the hand to the base of the thumb. (From Waldman S. *Atlas of Uncommon Pain
Syndromes*. 4th ed. Philadelphia: Elsevier; 2020 [Fig. 51-1].)

Cheiralgia paresthetica manifests as pain and associated paresthesias and
numbness of the radial aspect of the dorsum of the hand to the base of the thumb
(see Fig. 6.10). Because significant interpatient variability exists in the distribution
of the sensory branch of the radial nerve owing to overlap of the lateral antebrachial cutaneous nerve, the signs and symptoms of cheiralgia paresthetica may
vary from patient to patient.

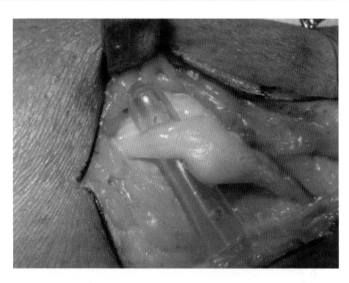

Fig. 6.10   Finding the neuroma on a dividing branch of the superficial branch of the radial nerve. (From Boussakri H, Reckendorf GMZ. Subcutaneous rupture of the superficial branch of the radial nerve at the wrist. A case report and review of literature. *Chirurgie de la Main*. 2015;34(3):141–144 [Fig. 2]. ISSN 1297-3203, https://doi.org/10.1016/j.main.2015.03.001, http://www.sciencedirect.com/science/article/pii/S1297320315000384.)

SIGNS AND SYMPTOMS

Physical findings include tenderness over the radial nerve at the wrist. A positive Tinel sign over the radial nerve at the distal forearm is usually present (see Fig. 6.1). Decreased sensation in the distribution of the sensory branch of the radial nerve is often present, although, as mentioned, the overlap of the lateral antebrachial cutaneous nerve may result in a confusing clinical presentation. A positive wristwatch sign also may be present (see Fig. 6.2). Flexion and pronation of the wrist and ulnar deviation often cause paresthesias in the distribution of the sensory branch of the radial nerve in patients with cheiralgia paresthetica.

TESTING

EMG can help identify the exact source of neurologic dysfunction and clarify the differential diagnosis; this should be the starting point of the evaluation of all patients thought to have cheiralgia paresthetica. Ultrasound evaluation of the radial nerve and its branches will help identify compression of the nerve from tumor, scar, hematoma, fracture, or other abnormalities (Fig. 6.11; see also Fig. 6.4). Plain radiographs are indicated in all patients who present with cheiralgia paresthetica to rule out occult bony pathologic processes. Based on the patient's clinical presentation, additional tests, including complete blood cell count, uric acid level, erythrocyte sedimentation rate, and antinuclear antibody testing, may be indicated. Magnetic

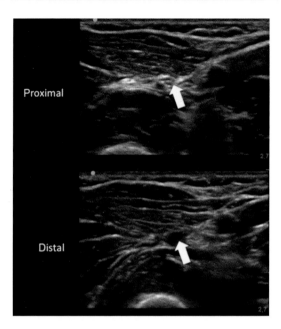

Fig. 6.11   Ultrasound images of the superficial branch of the radial nerve in the forearm above (cephalad to) a traumatic complete laceration of the nerve—a normal appearance proximally and a schwannoma in the edge of the nerve distally. Normal appearance proximally (*top arrow*) and a schwannoma in the edge of the nerve distally (*bottom arrow*). (From Tubbs R, Rizk E, Shoja M, et al. *Nerves and Nerve Injuries*. London: Academic Press; 2015 [Fig. 16-12].)

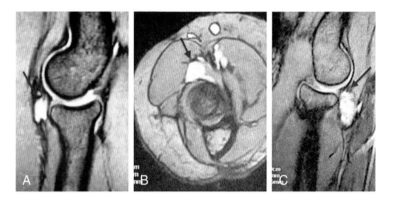

Fig. 6.12   (A) Sagital reconstruction of a MRI in T2 signal, showing a ganglion cyst coming from the radiocapitellar joint (red arrow). (B) Cross-section of a MRI in T2 signal showing a ganglion cyst anterior to the radial head (red arrow). (C) Sagital reconstruction of a MRI in T2 signal, showing a ganglion cyst coming from the radiocapitellar joint (red arrow). (From Miralles JR, Cisneros LN, Escola A, Fallone JC, Cots M, Espiga X. Type A ganglion cysts of the radiocapitellar joint may involve compression of the superficial radial nerve. *Orthopaedics & Traumatology: Surgery & Research*. 2016;102(6):791—796 [Fig. 1].)

resonance imaging (MRI) of the wrist is indicated if joint instability is suspected and to further clarify the pathology responsible for the patient's symptoms (Fig. 6.12). Injection of the sensory branch of the radial nerve at the wrist serves as a diagnostic and therapeutic maneuver and may be used as an anatomic differential neural blockade to distinguish lesions of the sensory branch of the radial nerve from lesions involving the lateral antebrachial cutaneous nerve.

DIFFERENTIAL DIAGNOSIS

Cheiralgia paresthetica is often misdiagnosed as lateral antebrachial cutaneous nerve syndrome. Cheiralgia paresthetica also should be differentiated

TABLE 6.1 ■ Causes of Compressive Radial Neuropathies

Site	Cause
High radial nerve	Trauma
	Fractures: Diaphyseal, distal third of the humerus
	Aneurysms
	Tumors
	Infection
	Inflammation: Local
	Anomalous muscles and arteries
	Idiopathic: Nerve torsion or localized constrictions
	Muscular effort: Lateral triceps
	Muscular hypertrophy
	Hereditary neuropathies
	External compression: Casts, crutches, braces, sleeping positions, tourniquets, walkers
Radial nerve	Radial tunnel: Pain without muscular weakness
	Anatomy: (1) Fibrous band, (2) vasculature leash (of Henry), (3) extensor carpi radialis brevis, (4) arcade of Frohse, (5) distal edge of supinator
	Musculature compression: Rowers, tennis players, weightlifters
	Metabolic: Pseudogout (joint swelling), rheumatoid arthritis
	Tumor: Synovial chondromatosis, ganglion, bicipital bursitis
	Infection: Septic arthritis
	External compression: Casts
Posterior interosseous nerve (PIN)	Same sites as the radial tunnel
	Surgical: Arthroscopy portals
	Tumor: Scapholunate ganglion, lipoma, intramuscular myxoma, ganglion
	Metabolic: Pseudogout
	Arteriovenous malformation, vasculitis
	Trauma: Dislocated radial head
	External compression: Casts, weight
	Idiopathic nerve constriction
Superficial branch	Wrist ganglion
	Anatomical: Fascia at brachoradialis/extensor carpi radialis brevis
	External compression: Casts, watch bands
	Crush injury

from cervical radiculopathy involving the C6 or C7 roots, although patients with cervical radiculopathy generally present not only with pain and numbness but also with reflex and motor changes. Cervical radiculopathy and radial nerve entrapment may coexist as the double crush syndrome. The double crush syndrome is seen most commonly with median nerve entrapment at the wrist or carpal tunnel syndrome. It should be remembered that radial nerve compression has many causes, and the nerve can be compressed anywhere along its path (Table 6.1).

TREATMENT

The first step in the treatment of cheiralgia paresthetica is the removal of the cause of pressure on the superficial radial nerve. A trial of nonsteroidal anti-inflammatory drugs or cyclooxyganse-2 inhibitors represents a reasonable next step. For patient for whom these treatment modalities fail, injection of the sensory branch of the radial nerve at the wrist should be considered. Ultrasound guidance may improve the accuracy of needle placement and decrease complications. For persistent symptoms, surgical exploration and decompression of the nerve are indicated.

HIGH-YIELD TAKEAWAYS

- The patient is afebrile, making an acute infectious etiology unlikely.
- The patient's symptomatology is thought to be the result of prolonged pressure on the right superficial radial nerve at the wrist from tight handcuffs.
- Physical examination and testing should be focused on the identification of the various causes of cheiralgia paresthetica.
- The patient exhibits the neurologic and physical examination findings that are highly suggestive of cheiralgia paresthetica.
- The patient's symptoms are unilateral suggestive of a local process rather than a systemic inflammatory process.
- Plain radiographs will provide high-yield information regarding the bony contents of the joint, but ultrasound imaging and MRI will be more useful in identifying soft tissue pathology that may be responsible for superficial radial nerve compromise at the wrist.
- EMG and nerve conduction velocity testing will help delineate the location and degree of nerve compromise if superficial radial nerve compromise is suspected.

Suggested Readings

Boussakri H, Reckendorf GMZ. Subcutaneous rupture of the superficial branch of the radial nerve at the wrist. A case report and review of literature. *Chirurgie de la Main*. 2015;34(3):141–144.

Helfenstein Jr M. Uncommon compressive neuropathies of upper limbs. *Best Pract Res Clin Rheumatol*. 2020;34(3):867–886.

Jordaan P, Wang CK, Ng CY. Management of painful cutaneous neuromas around the wrist. *Orthop Trauma*. 2017;31(4):290–295.

Waldman SD. Cheiralgia paresthetica. In: *Atlas of Uncommon Pain Syndromes*. 4th ed. Philadelphia: Elsevier; 2020:171–173.

Waldman SD. Cheiralgia paresthetica. In: *Pain Review*. 2nd ed. Philadelphia: Elsevier; 2017:260–261.

Waldman SD. Injection technique for radial nerve at the wrist. In: *Atlas of Interventional Pain Management*. 5th ed. Philadelphia: Elsevier; 2021:302–305.

Waldman SD. The wristwatch test for cheiralgia paresthetica. In: *Physical Diagnosis of Pain: An Atlas of Signs and Symptoms*. 4th ed. Philadelphia: Elsevier; 2021:185–186.

Waldman SD. Wartenberg syndrome and other disorders of the superficial radial nerve. In: *Waldman's Comprehensive Atlas of Diagnostic Ultrasound of Painful Conditions*. Philadelphia: Wolters Kluwer; 2016:399–406.

Mary Claire Bilman
A 68-Year-Old Female With Right Wrist Pain

- Learn the common causes of wrist pain.
- Develop an understanding of the unique anatomy of the carpometacarpal joints.
- Develop an understanding of the causes of arthritis of the carpometacarpal joints.
- Learn the clinical presentation of osteoarthritis of the carpometacarpal joints.
- Learn how to use physical examination to identify pathology associated with wrist pain.
- Develop an understanding of the treatment options for osteoarthritis of the carpometacarpal joints.
- Learn the appropriate testing options to help diagnose osteoarthritis of the carpometacarpal joints.
- Learn to identify red flags in patients who present with carpometacarpal joint pain.
- Develop an understanding of the role of interventional pain management in the treatment of carpometacarpal joint pain.

Mary Claire Bilman

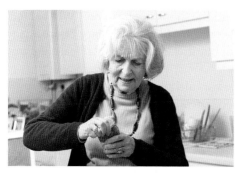

"Doctor, there is nothing golden about the golden years. Forty-some years of teaching, and I finally retire, and I immediately start falling apart! First the heart attack and now this. I have knitted my entire life. It's something that I really enjoy, and now it has become a real ordeal." Mary Claire Bilman was a longtime patient of mine, and I hated to see her so upset. Mary Claire is a 68-year-old retired kindergarten teacher with the chief complaint today of "I can't do my knitting anymore." She exclaims, "This wrist pain is really the pits. I can't brush my hair, and I am having to hold my toothbrush in my left hand." I asked if any of her other joints were bothering her, and she answered, "Just the usual aches and pains, but this right wrist is absolutely killing me. In all the years you have taken care of me, Doctor, have you ever heard me complain of pain? I don't believe in that pain stuff. I never said a thing about pain with my heart attack. If I hadn't been so dizzy, I wouldn't have even come in." I asked Mary Claire if she had experienced anything like this wrist pain in the past, before I started taking care of her, and she shook her head and responded, "Absolutely not. I can live with the aches and pains, it's just a part of growing old. I just toss down a couple of Tylenol with my evening glass of wine and leave it at that. But this time the reason I am here is right after dinner, I like to knit and watch the Home and Garden Network. If I can't knit, I am like a cat in a room full of rocking chairs. I can't seem to get settled down. Ever since my husband, Don, passed, the knitting is my friend, my companion." I asked, "Mary Claire, what about your cat?" "Harvey is in cat heaven," she replied, "and I have made a decision that I don't want anything else with DNA—no men, no dogs, no cats. Just fix my wrist so I can knit, and I won't bother you until my checkup next spring. And the other thing is, my wrist pain is waking me up at night. I've never been a good sleeper, but when I woke up at night, I would knit until I was able to get back to sleep. The golden years are really playing a joke on me with the wrist pain."

I asked Mary Claire about any antecedent trauma to the wrists, and she shook her head no. "Doctor, this wrist thing came out of nowhere! At first it wasn't that bad, and the Tylenol would take care of it. Now it hurts all the time. I can't open jars, tie my shoes, or hold my coffee cup. I can't even hold a pen to write a thank you note. I am in a real pickle here!"

I asked Mary Claire to point with one finger to show me where it hurts the most. She pointed to the base of her right thumb and said, "Doctor, it hurts worst here, but it also really hurts on the other side of my wrist by my little finger;

especially if I move my wrist toward the little finger when I use my right knitting needle to open up a stitch."

I asked if she had any fever or chills, and she shook her head no. "What about steroids? Did you ever take any cortisone or drugs like that?" Mary Claire again shook her head no. "I tried some Icy Hot but it was just too hot. Please get my wrist better, and I will knit you a hat."

On physical examination, Mary Claire was afebrile. Her respirations were 18 and her pulse was 70 and regular. Her blood pressure (BP) was 132/74. Her head, eyes, ears, nose, throat (HEENT) exam was normal, as was her cardiopulmonary exam. Her thyroid was normal. Her abdominal examination revealed no abnormal mass or organomegaly. There was no costovertebral angle (CVA) tenderness. There was no peripheral edema. Her low back examination was unremarkable. Visual inspection of the right wrist revealed no cutaneous lesions or obvious mass. The wrist was slightly warm to touch, but there was no obvious infection or swelling. Palpation of the right wrist revealed mild diffuse tenderness, with no obvious effusion. There was mild crepitus with range of motion. Range of motion of the carpometacarpal joints was decreased with pain exacerbated with flexion and extension of the wrist and especially with ulnar deviation. The Watson test was markedly positive on the right (Fig. 7.1). The left wrist examination was normal, as was examination of her other major joints, other than some mild osteoarthritis.

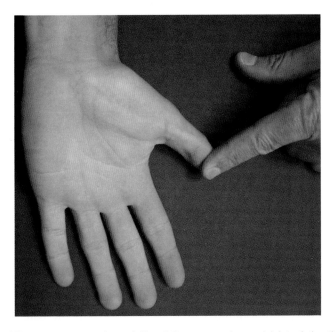

Fig. 7.1 The Watson stress test for arthritis of the carpometacarpal joint of the thumb. (From Waldman SD. *Physical Diagnosis of Pain*. 3rd ed. Philadelphia: Elsevier; 2016 [Fig. 106.2].)

A careful neurologic examination of the upper extremities revealed no evidence of peripheral or entrapment neuropathy, including carpal and ulnar tunnel syndromes. Deep tendon reflexes were normal.

Key Clinical Points—What's Important and What's Not

THE HISTORY

- No history of acute trauma
- No history of previous significant wrist pain
- No fever or chills
- Gradual onset of wrist pain with exacerbation of pain with wrist use
- Sleep disturbance
- Difficulty using the wrist to provide self-care and to knit

THE PHYSICAL EXAMINATION

- Patient is afebrile
- Normal visual inspection of wrist
- Palpation of right wrist reveals diffuse tenderness
- No point tenderness
- No increased temperature of right wrist
- Crepitus to palpation
- Watson test for arthritis of the carpometacarpal joint of the thumb was positive on the right (see Fig. 7.1)

OTHER FINDINGS OF NOTE

- Slightly elevated BP
- Normal HEENT examination
- Normal cardiovascular examination
- Normal pulmonary examination
- Normal abdominal examination
- No peripheral edema
- Normal upper extremity neurologic examination, motor and sensory examination
- Examination of other joints normal

 What Tests Would You Like to Order?

The following tests were ordered:
- Plain radiographs of the right wrist

TEST RESULTS

The plain radiographs of the right wrist revealed severe osteoarthritis of the carpometacarpal joints (Fig. 7.2).

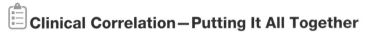 Clinical Correlation—Putting It All Together

What is the diagnosis?

- Osteoarthritis of the right wrist

The Science Behind the Diagnosis

ANATOMY OF THE WRIST JOINTS

The carpometacarpal joints of the fingers are synovium-lined ellipsoidal-type joints formed by the articular surface of the carpal bones proximally and the base

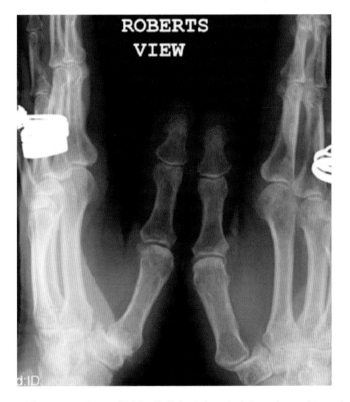

Fig. 7.2 X-ray of the carpometacarpal joint with Robert view depicting advanced trapeziometacarpal osteoarthritis. Subluxation of the first metacarpal bone has occurred. The severity of the malalignment is estimated by the hyperextension at the metacarpophalangeal joint. Osteophytes and sclerosis are present with joint space destruction.

of the second through fifth metacarpals distally (Fig. 7.3). The second metacarpal articulates primarily with the trapezoid and secondarily with the trapezium and capitate (see Fig. 7.3). The third metacarpal articulates primarily with the capitate, with the fourth metacarpal articulating with the capitate and hamate. The fifth metacarpal articulates with the hamate. The carpometacarpal joints of the fingers are shaped differently than the first carpometacarpal joint in that the curvature of the distal articular surface of the base of the metacarpal is more dome shaped, making for a more stable joint as it articulates with its corresponding

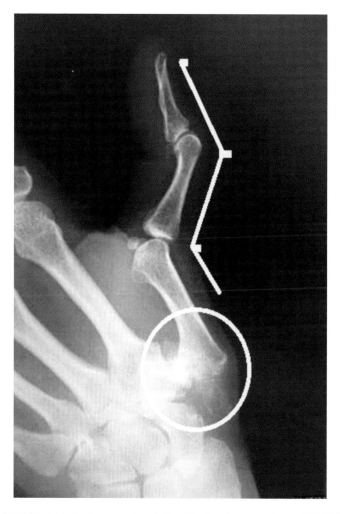

Fig. 7.3 Radiographic example of severe osteoarthritis of the thumb carpometacarpal (CMC) joint. The zigzag deformity, common in advanced stages of thumb CMC joint osteoarthritis, can be visualized. (From Grenier ML, Mendonca R, Dalley P. The effectiveness of orthoses in the conservative management of thumb CMC joint osteoarthritis: an analysis of functional pinch strength. *J Hand Ther.* 2016;29(3):307–313.)

carpal bones. Each joint is lined with synovium, and the ample synovial space allows for intraarticular placement of needles for injection and aspiration. Compared to the first carpometacarpal joint, the carpometacarpal joints of the fingers have a denser and tighter joint capsule and stronger transverse and interosseous ligaments. These differences combined with a much more limited range of motion when compared with the range of motion of the first carpometacarpal joint all contribute to greater joint stability, although fracture and subluxation still occur. The carpometacarpal joints of the fingers are also susceptible to overuse and misuse with resultant inflammation and arthritis.

THE CLINICAL SYNDROME

The carpometacarpal joints of the fingers are synovial plane joints that serve as the articulation between the carpals and the metacarpals and allow the bases of the metacarpal bones to articulate with one another. Movement of the joints is limited to a slight gliding motion, with the carpometacarpal joint of the little finger possessing the greatest range of motion. The primary function of these joints is to optimize the grip function of the hand. Most patients have a common joint space.

Pain and dysfunction from arthritis of the carpometacarpal joints are common complaints. These joints are susceptible to the development of arthritis from various conditions that share the ability to damage joint cartilage. Osteoarthritis is the most common form of arthritis that results in carpometacarpal joint pain (see Fig. 7.3). It occurs more often in female patients, and although the thumb is most frequently affected, arthritis may develop in the other carpometacarpal joints as well, especially after trauma. Rheumatoid arthritis, posttraumatic arthritis, and psoriatic arthritis are also common causes of carpometacarpal pain. Less frequent causes of arthritis-induced carpometacarpal pain include collagen vascular diseases, infection, and Lyme disease (Fig. 7.4). Acute infectious arthritis is usually accompanied by significant systemic symptoms, including fever and malaise, and should be easily recognized; it is treated with culture and antibiotics rather than injection therapy. Collagen vascular diseases generally manifest as polyarthropathy rather than as monarthropathy limited to the carpometacarpal joint; however, carpometacarpal pain secondary to collagen vascular disease responds exceedingly well to the intraarticular injection technique described here.

SIGNS AND SYMPTOMS

Most patients presenting with carpometacarpal pain secondary to osteoarthritis or posttraumatic arthritis complain of pain that is localized to the dorsum of the wrist. Activity associated with flexion, extension, and ulnar deviation of the carpometacarpal joints exacerbates the pain, whereas rest and heat provide some relief. The pain is constant and is characterized as aching; it may interfere with sleep.

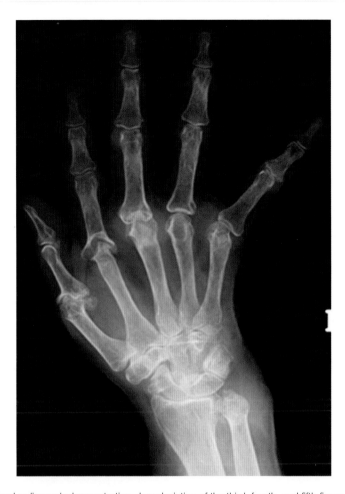

Fig. 7.4 Hand radiograph demonstrating ulnar deviation of the third, fourth, and fifth finger metacarpo-phalangeal (MCP) joints and pencil-and-cup deformity in the MCP joint of the first and second finger. (From Llopis E, Kroon HM, Acosta J, et al. Conventional radiology in rheumatoid arthritis. *Radiol Clin North Am*. 2017;55(5):917−941 [Fig. 17]. ISSN 0033-8389, ISBN 9780323545709, https://doi.org/10.1016/j.rcl.2017.04.002, http://www.sciencedirect.com/science/article/pii/S0033838917300489.)

Some patients complain of a grating or popping sensation with use of the joint, and crepitus may be present on physical examination. If the carpometacarpal joint of the thumb is affected, the patient will exhibit a positive Watson test. The test is performed by having the patient place the dorsum of the affected hand against a table with the fingers fully extended. The examiner then pushes the thumb toward the table. The test is positive if it reproduces the patient's pain (see Fig. 7.1).

In addition to pain, patients suffering from arthritis of the carpometacarpal joint often experience a gradual reduction in functional ability because of decreasing pinch and grip strength that makes everyday tasks such as using a pencil or opening a jar quite difficult. With continued disuse, muscle wasting may occur, and adhesive capsulitis with subsequent ankylosis may develop.

TESTING

Plain radiographs are indicated in all patients who present with carpometacarpal pain (Fig. 7.5). Based on the patient's clinical presentation, additional testing may be warranted, including a complete blood count, erythrocyte sedimentation rate, and antinuclear antibody testing. Magnetic resonance imaging (MRI) and ultrasound imaging of the affected carpometacarpal joint is indicated if joint instability is thought to be present, as well as to clarify the cause of joint pain and functional disability (Figs. 7.6 and 7.7). If infection is suspected, Gram stain and culture of the synovial fluid should be performed on an emergency basis, and treatment with appropriate antibiotics should be started. If the patient has a history of trauma, then computed tomography (CT), MRI, or radionuclide bone scanning may be useful because fractures of the navicular bone are often missed on plain radiographs of the wrist (Fig. 7.8).

DIFFERENTIAL DIAGNOSIS

Arthritis pain of the carpometacarpal joints is usually diagnosed on clinical grounds, and plain radiographs confirm the clinical findings (see Fig. 7.5).

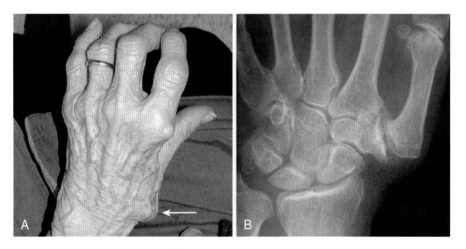

Fig. 7.5 First carpometacarpal arthritis. (A) Radial subluxation of the base of the first metacarpal giving the "shoulder sign" *(arrow)*. (B) Anteroposterior radiograph of the same hand. (From Young D, Papp S, Giachino A. Physical examination of the wrist. *Orthop Clin North Am.* 2007;38(2):149–165.)

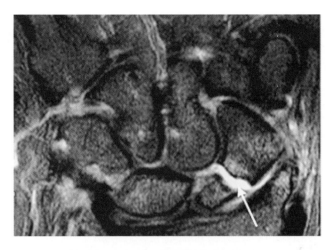

Fig. 7.6 Coronal long repetition time/echo time (TR/TE) fast spin-echo magnetic resonance image with fat saturation shows nonunion of a proximal pole scaphoid fracture *(arrow)*, outlined by fluid signal in the fracture. (From Edelman RR, Hesselink JR, Zlatkin MB, Crues JV, eds. *Clinical Magnetic Resonance Imaging.* 3rd ed. Philadelphia: Saunders; 2006:3344.)

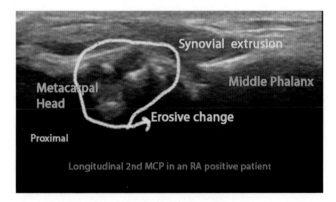

Fig. 7.7 Longitudinal ultrasound image demonstrating erosive changes of the second carpometacarpal joint. Note the synovial extrusion caused by exuberant synovitis. (From Waldman S. *Atlas of Common Pain Syndromes.* 4th ed. Philadelphia: Elsevier; 2019 [Fig. 53-3].)

Occasionally, arthritis pain of the carpometacarpal joints may be confused with de Quervain tenosynovitis or other forms of tendinitis involving the wrist and fingers. These painful conditions, as well as gout, may coexist and make the diagnosis more difficult. If the patient has a history of trauma, occult fractures of the metacarpals should always be considered (Table 7.1).

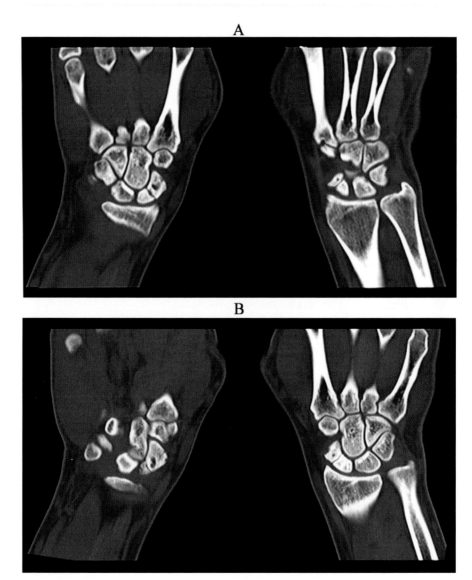

Fig. 7.8 A & B Computed tomography (CT) scan showing coronal views with bilateral scaphoid fractures. (From Kattan AE, Almarghoub MA, Alnujaim NH, et al. Bilateral scaphoid fractures: case report and literature review. *Int J Surg Case Rep.* 2020;66:412–415 [Fig. 2]. ISSN 2210-2612, https://doi.org/10.1016/j.ijscr.2020.01.005, http://www.sciencedirect.com/science/article/pii/S2210261220300146.)

TREATMENT

Initial treatment of the pain and functional disability associated with osteoarthritis of the carpometacarpal joints includes a combination of nonsteroidal antiinflammatory drugs (NSAIDs) or cyclooxygenase-2 inhibitors and physical

TABLE 7.1 ■ Causes of Wrist Pain

Bony Abnormalities

- Fracture
- Tumor
- Osteomyelitis
- Osteonecrosis
- Kienböck and Preiser diseases

Articular Abnormalities

- Osteoarthritis
- Rheumatoid arthritis

Collagen Vascular Diseases

- Reiter syndrome
- Psoriatic arthritis

Crystal Deposition Diseases

- Gout
- Pseudogout
- Pigmented villonodular synovitis
- Sprain
- Strain
- Hemarthrosis

Periarticular Abnormalities

- Tendon sheath disorders
- Trigger finger
- Flexor tenosynovitis
- Extensor tenosynovitis
- de Quervain tenosynovitis
- Dupuytren contracture
- Ganglion cyst
- Gouty tophi
- Subcutaneous nodules associated with rheumatoid arthritis
- Glomus tumor

Neurologic Abnormalities

- Median nerve entrapment
- Carpal tunnel syndrome
- Pronator syndrome
- Anterior interosseous nerve syndrome
- Ulnar nerve entrapment
- Ulnar tunnel syndrome
- Cubital tunnel syndrome
- Cheiralgia paresthetica
- Lower brachial plexus lesions
- Cervical nerve root lesions
- Spinal cord lesions
- Syringomyelia
- Spinal cord tumors
- Reflex sympathetic dystrophy
- Causalgia

(Continued)

TABLE 7.1 ■ Causes of Wrist Pain—cont'd

Vascular Abnormalities
- Vasculitis
- Raynaud syndrome
- Takayasu arteritis
- Scleroderma

Referred Pain
- Shoulder-hand syndrome
- Angina

From Waldman S. *Physical Diagnosis of Pain: An Atlas of Signs and Symptoms*. 4th ed. Philadelphia: Elsevier; 2021 (table 113–1).

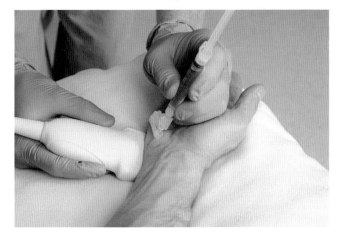

Fig. 7.9   Proper needle position for ultrasound-guided out-of-plane injection of the carpometacarpal joints of the fingers joint.

therapy. Local application of heat and cold may also be beneficial. Splinting the wrist in the neutral position may provide symptomatic relief and protect the joint from additional trauma. For patients who do not respond to these treatment modalities, intraarticular injection of local anesthetic and steroid is a reasonable next step. Ultrasound guidance will increase the accuracy of needle placement and decrease the incidence of needle-induced complications (Fig. 7.9). Clinical experience has suggested that injection of platelet-rich plasma and/or stem cells may hasten resolution of the patient's joint symptomatology. Ultrasound needle guidance will aid in accurate needle placement.

HIGH-YIELD TAKEAWAYS

- The patient is afebrile, making an acute infectious etiology (e.g., septic arthritis) unlikely.
- The patient's symptomatology is not the result of acute trauma but more likely the result of repetitive microtrauma that has damaged the joint over time.
- The patient's pain is more diffuse rather than highly localized as would be the case with a pathologic process such as fracture or de Quervain tenosynovitis.
- The patient's symptoms are unilateral and involve only one joint, which is more suggestive of a local process than a systemic polyarthropathy.
- Sleep disturbance is common and must be addressed concurrently with the patient's pain symptomatology.
- Plain radiographs will provide high-yield information regarding the bony contents of the joint, but ultrasound imaging and MRI will be more useful in identifying soft tissue pathology.

Suggested Readings

Bay COA, Willacy RA, Moses AR, et al. Nonspecific wrist pain in pediatric patients: a systematic review. *J Orthop.* 2020;22:308–315.

Brewer PE, Storey PA. The hand and wrist in rheumatoid and osteoarthritis. *Surgery (Oxford).* 2016;34(3):144–151.

Dineen HA, Greenberg JA. Ulnar-sided wrist pain in the athlete. *Clin Sport Med.* 2020;39(2):373–400.

Islam SUl, Brown D, Cheung G. Management of osteoarthritis of the wrist and hand. *Orthop Trauma.* 2019;33(1):30–37.

Laulan J, Marteau E, Bacle G. Wrist osteoarthritis. *Orthop Traumatol Surg Res.* 2015;101(1):S1–S9.

Waldman SD. Abnormalities of the distal radioulnar joint. In: *Waldman's Comprehensive Atlas of Diagnostic Ultrasound of Painful Conditions.* Philadelphia: Wolters Kluwer; 2016:353–360.

Waldman SD. Arthritis and other disorders of the carpometacarpal joints of the fingers. In: *Waldman's Comprehensive Atlas of Diagnostic Ultrasound of Painful Conditions.* Philadelphia: Wolters Kluwer; 2016:446–450.

Waldman SD. Functional anatomy of the wrist. In: *Physical Diagnosis of Pain: An Atlas of Signs and Symptoms.* 3rd ed Philadelphia: Saunders; 2016:158–159.

Waldman SD. Intra-articular injection of the carpometacarpal joint. In: *Atlas of Pain Management Injection Techniques.* 4th ed. Philadelphia: Elsevier; 2017:290–293.

Waldman SD. The Watson stress test for arthritis of the carpometacarpal joint of the thumb. In: *Physical Diagnosis of Pain: An Atlas of Signs and Symptoms.* 3rd ed. Elsevier; 2016:173–174.

Waldman SD. Arthritis pain at the carpometacarpal joints. In: *Atlas of Common Pain Syndromes.* 4th ed. Elsevier; 2019:208–211.

Jessie Bumgartner

A 64-Year-Old Homemaker With Left Wrist Pain and Swelling

- Learn the common causes of wrist pain.
- Develop an understanding of the unique anatomy of the wrist joint.
- Develop an understanding of the characteristics of ganglion cysts.
- Develop an understanding of the causes of ganglion cysts.
- Develop an understanding of the differential diagnosis of ganglion cysts.
- Learn the clinical presentation of ganglion cysts.
- Learn how to examine the wrist.
- Learn how to use physical examination to identify ganglion cysts.
- Develop an understanding of the treatment options for ganglion cysts.

Jessie Bumgartner

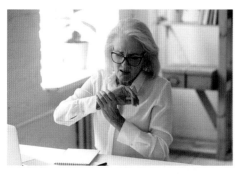

Jessie Bumgartner is a 64-year-old homemaker with the chief complaint of "I've got a bump on my wrist and it won't go away." Jessie stated that over the past several months her right wrist started "swelling up like a balloon." She went on to say, "This is so embarrassing! I always had pretty hands." I asked Jessie if she ever had anything like this before, and she said, "Are you kidding? Look at this! Doctor, do you know what a manitou is? Because that is what this is beginning to look like." I responded, "You mean the Canadian province Manitoba?" She laughed, then said, "No, Doctor, a manitou." I replied, "Jessie, you got me there. Tell me what a manitou is." She said, "Doctor, you need to up your game here. A manitou is a spiritual being that returns to this world and grows on a living being. It's an old Native American legend, and that is just what this looks like." I let that sink in for a minute, and then said, "So you think a spirit is growing in that lump on your wrist?" Jessie laughed again and said, "Well, unless you have a better idea, I am stuck with a manitou. But whatever it is, it's certainly getting bigger, and it hurts when I move my wrist. This is really not the look I am going for now that I am back on the dating scene. My manitou is not going to help me on eHarmony!"

I asked Jessie what made her wrist pain worse, and she said that any movement of the wrist, especially flexion, caused pain. "Doctor, I can live with the pain, but the look is really not working for me. This is really embarrassing—nothing Botox or fillers are going to fix." I asked her what made the pain better, and she said Advil seemed to help the pain but not the swelling, but the Advil was upsetting her stomach. She noted that the heating pad felt good, but she thought it made her wrist swell more. "I also tried using an Ace wrap, but I felt like it was cutting off my circulation." I asked Jessie about any antecedent wrist trauma, and she said, "Not that I can remember."

I asked Jessie to point with one finger to show me where it hurt the most. She pointed to one of the largest ganglion cysts I had ever seen. She really wasn't kidding when she said the wrist had something growing on it. It literally was no exaggeration. "So this is what a manitou looks like?" I asked (Fig. 8.1).

On physical examination, Jessie was afebrile. Her respirations were 16 and her pulse was 74 and regular. Her blood pressure was 126/76. Jessie's head, eyes, ears, nose, throat (HEENT) exam was normal, as was her cardiopulmonary examination. Her thyroid was normal. Her abdominal examination revealed no abnormal mass or organomegaly. There was no costovertebral angle (CVA)

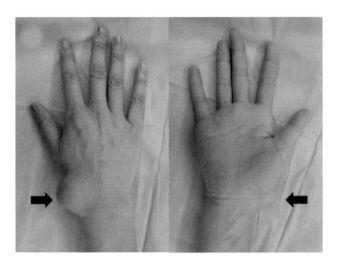

Fig. 8.1   Large dorsal ganglion cyst of the right wrist. (From Yamamoto M, Kurimoto S, Okui N, et al. Sonography-assisted arthroscopic resection of volar wrist ganglia: a new technique. *Arthr Tech.* 2012;1(1):e31—e35 [Fig. 1A]. ISSN 2212-6287, https://doi.org/10.1016/j.eats.2011.12.007, http://www .sciencedirect.com/science/article/pii/S2212628712000102.)

tenderness. There was no peripheral edema. Her low back examination revealed some tenderness to deep palpation of the paraspinous musculature. Visual inspection of the right wrist revealed a huge dorsal ganglion cyst (see Fig. 8.1). The cyst transilluminated with a penlight, effectively ruling out a solid tumor. There was a positive ganglion cyst extreme flexion extension test with a marked increase in pain with extreme flexion of the wrist (Fig. 8.2). Range of motion of the wrist joint, especially resisted extension and passive flexion of the wrist joint, caused Jessie to cry out in pain. The left wrist examination was normal, as was examination of her major joints. A careful neurologic examination of the upper and lower extremities revealed there was no evidence of peripheral or entrapment neuropathy, and the deep tendon reflexes were normal.

Key Clinical Points—What's Important and What's Not

THE HISTORY

- Gradual onset of a mass on the dorsum of her right wrist
- Pain with flexion and extension of the wrist
- Significant concern regarding the cosmetic impact of the wrist
- Pain made worse with extreme flexion of the wrist
- No other specific traumatic event to the area identified
- No fever or chills

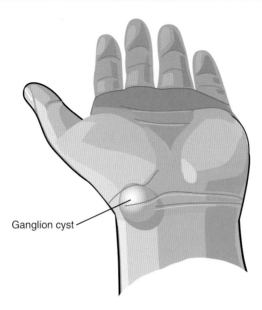

Ganglion cyst

Fig. 8.2   The extreme flexion/extension test for ganglion cyst of the wrist. To perform the extreme flex-ion/extension test for ganglion cyst of the wrist, the examiner first localizes the ganglion cyst to the dorsal or volar aspect of the wrist. If the ganglion is on the dorsal aspect, the examiner forcefully flexes the patient's affected wrist. If the ganglion cyst is located on the volar aspect of the wrist, the examiner forcefully extends the patient's affected wrist *(see illustration)*. The extreme flexion/extension test is positive if the forceful flexion or extension of the wrist causes a marked increase in the patient's pain. (From Waldman S. *Physical Diagnosis of Pain: An Atlas of Signs and Symptoms*. 4th ed. Philadelphia: Elsevier; 2021 [Fig. 129.2].)

THE PHYSICAL EXAMINATION

- Patient is afebrile
- Large mass on the dorsum of the right wrist
- Wrist mass transilluminates
- No evidence of infection
- Pain on range of motion, especially extreme flexion of the affected right wrist
- The extreme flexion/extension test for ganglion cyst of the wrist was positive on the right (see Fig. 8.2)

OHER FINDINGS OF NOTE

- Normal HEENT examination
- Normal cardiovascular examination
- Normal pulmonary examination
- Normal abdominal examination

- No tenderness to deep palpation of the lumbar paraspinous muscles
- No peripheral edema
- Normal upper and lower extremity neurologic examination, motor and sensory examination
- Examination of joints other than the right wrist was normal

What Tests Would You Like to Order?

The following tests were ordered:
- Ultrasound of the left wrist

TEST RESULTS

Ultrasound examination of the left wrist revealed a large dorsal ganglion cyst of the wrist (Fig. 8.3).

Clinical Correlation—Putting It All Together

What is the diagnosis?
- Dorsal ganglion cyst of the wrist

The Science Behind the Diagnosis

ANATOMY

The dorsum of the wrist is especially susceptible to the development of ganglion cysts in the area overlying the extensor tendons or the joint space, with a predilection for the joint space of the lunate or from the tendon sheath of the extensor carpi radialis (Fig. 8.4; see also Fig. 8.1). The volar aspect of the wrist can also be affected.

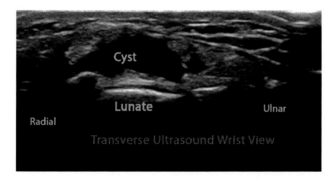

Fig. 8.3 Ultrasound image of a large dorsal ganglion cyst of the wrist. (From Waldman S. *Atlas of Common Pain Syndromes*. 4th ed. Philadelphia: Elsevier; 2019 [Fig. 54-6].)

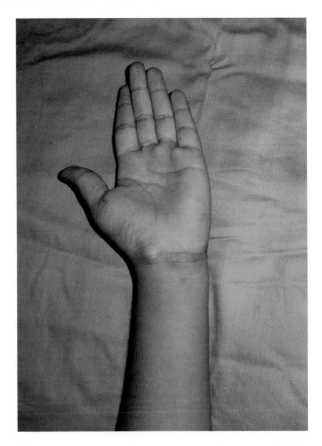

Fig. 8.4 Ganglion cyst of the volar wrist. (From Chaudhary S, Mandal S, Kumar V. Results of modified thread technique for the treatment of wrist ganglion. *J Clin Orthop Trauma*. 2020 [Fig. 1]. ISSN 0976-5662, https://doi.org/10.1016/j.jcot.2020.08.018, http://www.sciencedirect.com/science/article/pii/S0976566220304033.)

CLINICAL SYNDROME

Ganglion cysts are thought to form as the result of herniation of synovial-containing tissues from joint capsules or tendon sheaths. This tissue may then become irritated and begin producing increased amounts of synovial fluid, which can pool in cystlike cavities overlying the tendons and joint space. A one-way valve phenomenon may cause these cystlike cavities to expand because the fluid cannot flow freely back into the synovial cavity. Ganglion cysts occur most commonly on the dorsal aspect of the wrist but may also occur on the volar aspect of the wrist (Figs. 8.5 and 8.6). Occurring three times more commonly in women than in men, ganglion cysts of the wrist represent 65% to 70% of all soft tissue tumors of the hand and wrist. Ganglion cysts occur in all age groups, with a peak incidence in fourth to sixth decades.

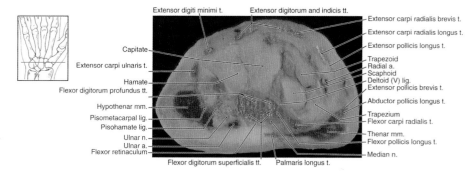

Fig. 8.5 Ganglion cysts of the wrists are thought to form as the result of herniation of synovial-containing tissues from joint capsules or tendon sheaths. (From Kang HS, Ahn JM, Resnick D. *MRI of the Extremities: An Anatomic Atlas*. 2nd ed. Philadelphia: Saunders; 2002:178.)

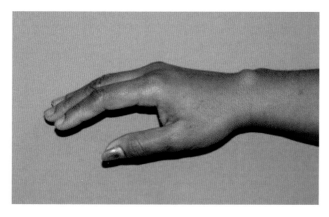

Fig. 8.6 A typical dorsal ganglion cyst. (From Waldman S. *Atlas of Common Pain Syndromes*. 4th ed. Philadelphia: Elsevier; 2019 [Fig. 54-2].)

SIGNS AND SYMPTOMS

Activity, especially extreme flexion and extension, makes the pain worse; rest and heat provide some relief. The pain is constant and is characterized as aching. Occasionally, the ganglion will cause a trigger wrist. Often, the unsightly nature of the ganglion cyst, rather than the pain, causes the patient to seek medical attention (Fig. 8.7). The ganglion is smooth to palpation and transilluminates with a penlight, in contradistinction to solid tumors, which do not transilluminate. Palpation of the ganglion may increase the pain.

TESTING

Plain radiographs of the wrist are indicated in all patients who present with ganglion cysts to rule out bony abnormalities, including tumors (Fig. 8.8).

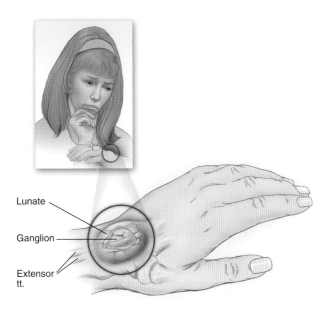

Fig. 8.7   Ganglion cysts usually appear on the dorsum of the wrist, overlying the extensor tendon or joint space. Patients often seek medical attention out of a fear of cancer. (From Waldman S. *Atlas of Common Pain Syndromes*. 4th ed. Philadelphia: Elsevier; 2019 [Fig. 54-3].)

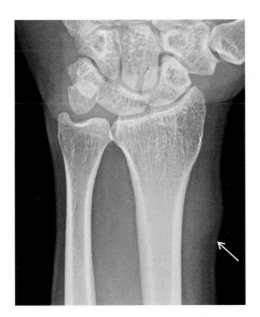

Fig. 8.8   Anteroposterior radiograph of the left wrist showing a focal soft tissue prominence on the radial side *(arrow)* with no mineralization or underlying bony involvement. (From Weeks JK, Strauch RJ, Virk RK, et al. Cephalic venous aneurysm in the wrist. *Clin Imaging*. 2018;52:310—314 [Fig. 2]. ISSN 0899-7071, https://doi.org/10.1016/j.clinimag.2018.07.001, http://www.sciencedirect.com/science/article/pii/S0899707118301906.)

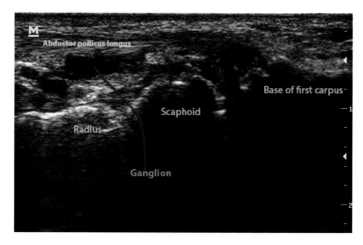

Fig. 8.9   Longitudinal ultrasound image demonstrating a ganglion cyst of the wrist lying beneath the abductor pollicis longus.

Ultrasound imaging will help determine whether a soft tissue mass of the wrist is cystic or solid (Fig. 8.9). Based on the patient's clinical presentation, additional testing may be indicated, including complete blood count, sedimentation rate, and antinuclear antibody testing. Magnetic resonance imaging (MRI) and ultrasound imaging of the wrist are indicated if the cause of the wrist mass is suspect (Figs. 8.10 and 8.11).

DIFFERENTIAL DIAGNOSIS

Although ganglion cysts are the most common soft tissue tumor of the wrist, many other pathologic processes can mimic this disorder (Box 8.1). Infection, tenosynovitis, lipomas, and carpal bosses are among the more common diseases that may mimic ganglion cysts of the wrist. Less commonly, malignant tumors, including sarcomas, and metastatic disease may confuse the diagnosis (Fig. 8.12).

TREATMENT

Initial treatment of the pain and functional disability associated with ganglion cyst of the wrist includes a combination of nonsteroidal antiinflammatory drugs or cyclooxygenase-2 inhibitors and physical therapy. Local application of heat and cold may also be beneficial. Splinting the wrist in the neutral position may provide symptomatic relief and protect the joint from additional trauma. For patients who do not respond to these treatment modalities, injection of the ganglion cyst with local anesthetic and steroid is a reasonable next step (Fig. 8.13).

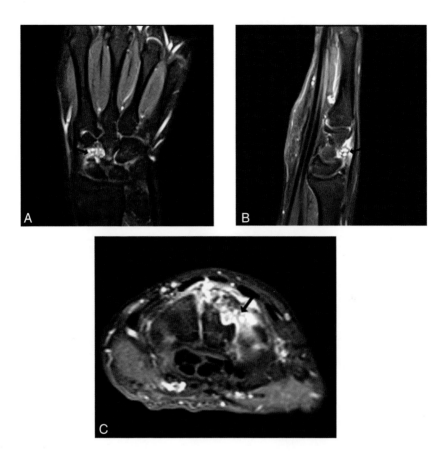

Fig. 8.10 (A, B, C) Magnetic resonance imaging showing three views of a synovial hemangioma mimicking a dorsal ganglion cyst. (From Zhao X, Qi C, Chen J, et al. Synovial hemangioma of the wrist with cystic invasion of trapezoid and capitate bones. *J Hand Surg.* 2020;45(2):161.e1–161.e6 [Fig. 2]. ISSN 0363-5023, https://doi.org/10.1016/j.jhsa.2019.03.007, http://www.sciencedirect.com/science/article/pii/S0363502318303162.)

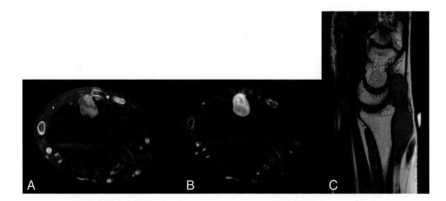

Fig. 8.11 Magnetic resonance imaging (MRI) of the wrist mass. (A) A fat-suppressed T1 and (B) T2 MRI demonstrate a mass emerging between the third and fourth dorsal compartments. (C) Sagittal MRI illustrates the dumbbell-shaped appearance of the intraneural neurofibroma of the posterior interosseous nerve. (From Gandhi RA, Bozentka DJ. Bilateral plexiform neurofibromas of the posterior interosseous nerve mimicking dorsal wrist ganglions. *J Hand Surg.* 2020;45(8):781.e1–781.e4 [Fig. 1]. ISSN 0363-5023, https://doi.org/10.1016/j.jhsa.2019.10.016, http://www.sciencedirect.com/science/article/pii/S0363502319314285.)

BOX 8.1 ■ Diseases That May Mimic Ganglion Cyst of the Wrist

- Infection
- Lipoma
- Tenosynovitis
- Carpal boss
- Neuroma
- Hypertrophied extensor digitorum brevis manus muscle belly
- Instability of the scaphoid
- Instability of the lunate
- Scaphotrapezial arthritis
- Vascular aneurysm
- Sarcoma

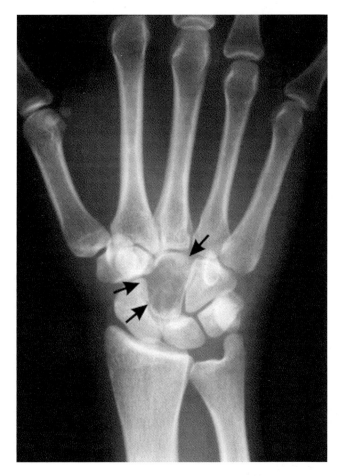

Fig. 8.12 Posteroanterior radiograph of the right hand in a patient thought to have a dorsal ganglion cyst of the wrist demonstrating a lytic lesion of the *capitate* (*arrows*) with cortical destruction secondary to metastatic malignant melanoma. (From Tomas X, Conill C, Combalia A, *et al*. Malignant melanoma with metastasis into the capitate. *Eur J Radiol*. 2005;56(3):362–364.)

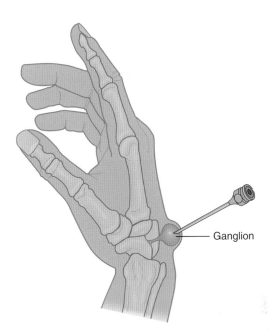

Fig. 8.13 Injection technique for the treatment of ganglion cysts of the wrist. (From Waldman SD. *Atlas of Pain Management Injection Techniques.* 2nd ed. Philadelphia: Saunders; 2007:273.)

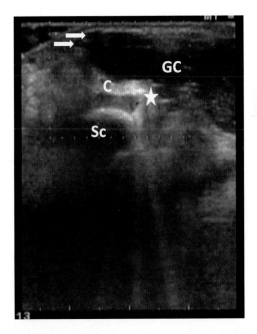

Fig. 8.14 Ultrasound-guided arthroscopic excision of a ganglion cyst of the wrist. Color Doppler sonography shows the branches of the radial artery *(arrows)*. The tip of the arthroscopic shaver *(star)* is clearly visible with an acoustic shadow during shaving. *C*, Radiocarpal joint capsule; *GC*, ganglion cyst; *Sc*, scaphoid. (From Yamamoto M, Kurimoto S, Okui N, et al. Sonography-assisted arthroscopic resection of volar wrist ganglia: a new technique. *Arthr Tech.* 2012;1(1):e31–e35 [Fig. 3]. ISSN 2212-6287, https://doi.org/10.1016/j.eats.2011.12.007, http://www.sciencedirect.com/science/article/pii/S2212628712000102.)

If symptoms persist, surgical excision of the ganglion is recommended (Fig. 8.14). Other treatment options include placing a large sterile surgical suture through the ganglion with the suture left in place as a drain for several days (Figs. 8.15 and 8.16).

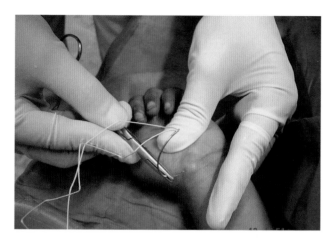

Fig. 8.15   The thread technique for the treatment of ganglion cyst. Clinical photograph showing thread on a cutting needle being passed through a ganglion cyst of the volar wrist. (From Chaudhary S, Mandal S, Kumar V. Results of modified thread technique for the treatment of wrist ganglion. *J Clin Orthop Trauma*. 2020 [Fig. 2]. ISSN 0976-5662, https://doi.org/10.1016/j.jcot.2020.08.018, http://www.sciencedirect.com/science/article/pii/S0976566220304033.)

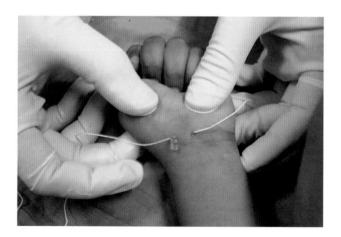

Fig. 8.16   Mucinous ganglion contents being expressed out around the previously placed thread. (From Chaudhary S, Mandal S, Kumar V. Results of modified thread technique for the treatment of wrist ganglion. *J Clin Orthop Trauma*. 2020 [Fig. 3]. ISSN 0976-5662, https://doi.org/10.1016/j.jcot.2020.08.018, http://www.sciencedirect.com/science/article/pii/S0976566220304033.)

HIGH-YIELD TAKEAWAYS

- The patient is afebrile, making an acute infectious etiology (e.g., septic arthritis) unlikely.

- The patient's symptomatology is highly suggestive of a ganglion cyst, and physical examination and testing should be focused on the identification of ligamentous injury, acute arthritis, tendinitis, and bursitis that may also be contributing to the patient's pain symptomatology as ganglion cysts may impinge on other anatomic structures.

- The patient's mass transilluminates, which is highly suggestive of a cystic mass, most likely a ganglion cyst.

- The patient's symptoms are unilateral and involve only one joint, which is more suggestive of a local process than a systemic polyarthropathy.

- Ultrasound imaging is highly specific in the diagnosis of ganglion cysts.

- Plain radiographs will provide high-yield information regarding the bony contents of the joint and the identification of fractures or other bony abnormalities of the femur as well as calcification of the bursa and tendons.

- Ultrasound imaging and MRI will be more useful in identifying soft tissue pathology that may be mimicking the clinical presentation of ganglion cyst of the wrist.

Suggested Readings

Al-Qattan MM, Elshamma NA, Alqabbani A. Trigger wrist and carpal tunnel syndrome caused by a flexor tendon-related ganglion in a teenager: a case report. *Int J Surg Case Rep.* 2017;30:86–88.

Balazs GC, Dworak TC, Tropf J, et al. Incidence and risk factors for volar wrist ganglia in the US military and civilian populations. *J Hand Surg Am.* 2016;41(11):1064–1070.

Head L, Gencarelli JR, Allen M, et al. Wrist ganglion treatment: systematic review and meta-analysis. *J Hand Surg Am.* 2015;40(3):546–553, e8.

Waldman SD. Ganglion cysts of the wrist. In: *Atlas of Common Pain Syndromes.* 4th ed. Philadelphia: Elsevier; 2018:212–216.

Waldman SD. Ganglion cysts of the wrist. In: *Waldman's Comprehensive Atlas of Diagnostic Ultrasound of Painful Conditions.* Philadelphia: Wolters Kluwer; 2016:432–438.

Waldman SD. Injection technique for ganglion cysts of the wrist and hand. In: *Atlas of Pain Management Injection Techniques.* 4th ed. Philadelphia: Elsevier; 2017:322–324.

Waldman SD, Campbell RSD. Ganglion cyst of the wrist. In: *Imaging of Pain.* Philadelphia: Saunders; 2011:327–329.

CHAPTER
9

Bobby Marcelo

A 48-Year-Old Male With a Painful Bump on the Back of His Wrist

Bobby Marcelo

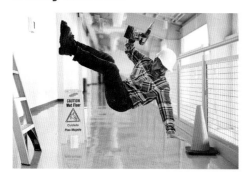

Bobby Marcelo is a 48-year-old electrician with the chief complaint of "I have a painful bump on the back of my wrist ever since I fell off my ladder." Bobby stated that a couple of months ago, as he was installing a smoke detector, he missed a step on his ladder and fell backward and landed on his outstretched hand. He said, "God was with me that day. I could have broken my neck." Bobby said that he was "pretty shook up," but once he realized that he wasn't badly hurt, he got up and went back to work. "Doc, with all of the layoffs, I decided to just keep my mouth shut about my fall. I went home and iced my wrist and had a couple of cold ones, took some Advil, and went to bed." Bobby went on to say that over the next month, he began to notice a bump on the back of his right wrist. "Doc, this thing really scared me. You know that my dad died of prostate cancer? It spread to his bones. You don't think that's what it is, do you?" I told Bobby that I had no reason to suspect that the bump on his wrist was cancer, but I would be sure to keep this in mind as we worked together to sort out what the bump was. "Doc, I can't believe I fell off my ladder! This has never happened in all the years I have been an electrician. I am really careful!"

I asked Bobby if he had experienced any pain, numbness, or weakness in his hand since the fall, and he shook his head and replied, "Never. Doc, the pain is around the bump, and it can hurt when I move my wrist. I can live with the pain. I just don't want the cancer. Oh, and if you push on the bump—oh boy! The pain gets a lot worse." I asked Bobby how he was sleeping, and he said, "Not worth a crap, Doc. Every time I roll over, if I move my wrist, the pain wakes me up. And the worry about what this bump is hasn't helped."

I asked Bobby to show me where the pain was, and he pointed to the bump on the dorsum of his wrist. "Doc, the pain is right around this bump; that's where the pain is." I asked, "Does the pain radiate anywhere?" Bobby shook his head and said, "Doc, let's not worry about the pain. Let's just figure out whether or not I have cancer." I reassured Bobby that I was taking this very seriously and all of these questions were to help me figure out what was causing the bump. I asked Bobby about any fever, chills, or other constitutional symptoms such as weight loss, night sweats, etc., and he shook his head no. He denied any musculoskeletal, systemic symptoms, or bowel or bladder symptoms.

On physical examination, Bobby was afebrile. His respirations were 18, his pulse was 72 and regular, and his blood pressure was 124/76. Bobby's head, eyes, ears, nose, throat (HEENT) exam was normal, as was his thyroid exam. Auscultation of his carotids revealed no bruits, and the pulses in all four extremities were normal. He had a regular rhythm without ectopy. His cardiac exam was otherwise unremarkable. His abdominal examination revealed no abnormal mass or organomegaly. There was no peripheral edema. His low back examination was unremarkable. There was no costovertebral angle (CVA) tenderness. I did a rectal exam, which revealed a completely normal prostate. Visual inspection of the right wrist revealed a firm, unmovable mass on the dorsum of the wrist (Fig. 9.1). The mass did not transilluminate with my penlight, suggesting that this was not a cystic mass like a dorsal ganglion cyst. There was no rubor or color and no evidence of ecchymosis of the skin overlying the mass. Deep palpation of the mass elicited pain, as did extreme flexion of the right wrist. There was no other obvious bony deformity that would suggest a previous fracture. The hunchback carpal sign was positive on the right (Fig. 9.2). The Allen test was normal bilaterally, as were the Phalen and Tinel tests for carpal tunnel syndrome. The left wrist examination was completely normal, as was examination of Bobby's other joints. A careful neurologic examination of both lower extremities was within normal limits. Deep tendon reflexes were physiologic throughout.

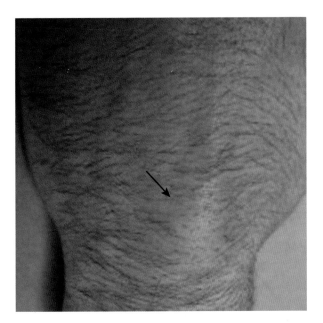

Fig. 9.1 The carpal boss is frequently confused initially with a dorsal ganglion on viewing the dorsal wrist. It generally feels harder with palpation, is positioned more distally than wrist ganglion, and overlies the index and middle finger carpometacarpal joints *(arrow)*. (From Park MJ, Namdari S, Weiss AP. The carpal boss: review of diagnosis and treatment. *J Hand Surg.* 2008;33(3):446−449.)

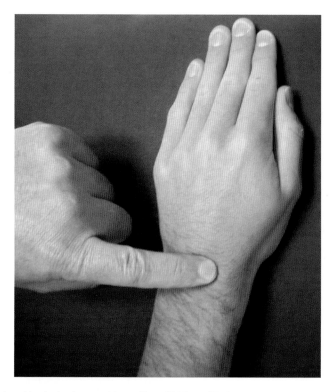

Fig. 9.2 The hunchback sign for carpal boss. (From Waldman SD. Painful conditions of the wrist and hand. In: *Physical diagnosis of pain: an atlas of signs and symptoms*. 2nd ed. Philadelphia: Saunders; 2010:189.)

Key Clinical Points—What's Important and What's Not

THE HISTORY

- A history of right wrist pain immediately following a fall from a ladder
- The gradual appearance of a mass on the dorsum of the wrist
- The patient's chief concern is that he has cancer
- The pain is localized to the wrist and no other joints
- Use of the wrist can exacerbate the pain
- There is significant sleep disturbance
- No fever or chills

THE PHYSICAL EXAMINATION

- Patient is afebrile
- Firm unmovable mass on the dorsum of the right wrist
- Marked tenderness to palpation of the wrist mass
- Marked pain with extreme flexion of the wrist

- Positive carpal hunchback test (see Fig. 9.2)
- Mass did not transilluminate
- Normal neurologic examination, specifically no signs of carpal tunnel syndrome

OTHER FINDINGS OF NOTE

- Normal HEENT examination
- Normal cardiovascular examination
- Normal pulmonary examination
- Normal abdominal examination
- Negative Allen test
- No peripheral edema

 ## What Tests Would You Like to Order?

The following tests were ordered:
- X-ray of the wrist

TEST RESULTS

X-ray of the wrist reveals a carpal boss at the base of the third metacarpal and capitate (Fig. 9.3).

 ## Clinical Correlation—Putting It All Together

What is the diagnosis?
- Carpal boss

The Science Behind the Diagnosis

CLINICAL SYNDROME

Carpal boss syndrome, or os styloideum, is characterized by localized tenderness and sharp pain over the junction of the second and third carpometacarpal joints. The pain of carpal boss syndrome results from exostosis of the second and third carpometacarpal joints or, more uncommonly, a loose body involving the intraarticular space (Fig. 9.4). Patients often report that the pain is worse after rigorous physical activity involving the hand rather than during the activity itself. The pain of carpal boss syndrome may also radiate locally, thus confusing the clinical presentation. The disease typically affects the dominant hand, although carpal bossing is present approximately 15% of the time in patients suffering

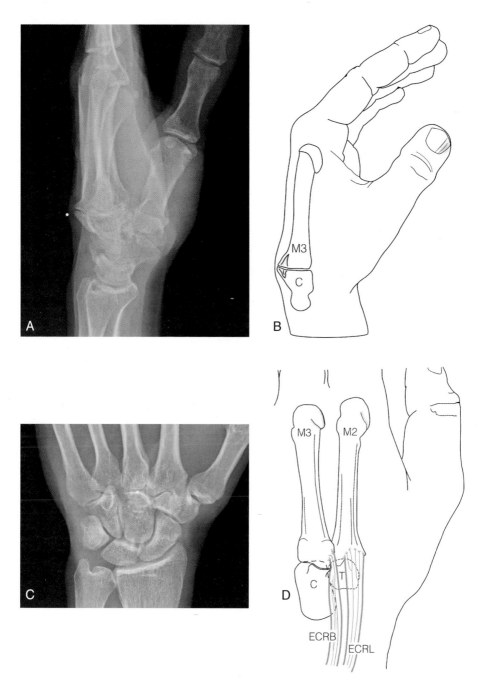

Fig. 9.3 Lateral radiograph (A) metallic marker and (B) diagram demonstrate a carpal boss at the base of the third metacarpal and capitate. Frontal radiograph (C) metallic marker and (D) diagram demonstrate the carpal boss and a theoretic depiction of associated displacement of the extensor carpi radialis brevis tendon. *C,* Capitate; *ECRB,* extensor carpi radialis brevis; *ECRL,* extensor carpi radialis longus; *M2,* second metacarpal; *M3,* third metacarpal; *T,* trapezoid. (From Porrino J, Maloney E, Chew FS. Current concepts of the carpal boss: pathophysiology, symptoms, clinical or imaging diagnosis, and management. *Curr Prob Diag Radiol.* 2015;44(5):462–468 [Fig. 1]. ISSN 0363-0188, https://doi.org/10.1067/j.cpradiol.2015.02.008, http://www.sciencedirect.com/science/article/pii/S0363018815000274.)

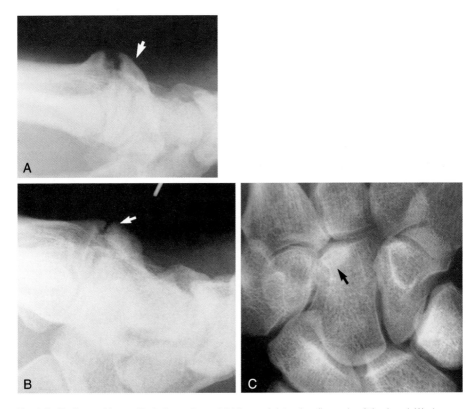

Fig. 9.4   Radiographic manifestations of os styloideum. A lateral radiograph of the hand (A) demonstrates the osteophytic appearance of the extra ossification center *(arrow)*. Clinically, a painless soft tissue lump is often evident. In another patient, a similar outgrowth *(arrows)* is evident on lateral (B) and frontal (C) radiographs. (From Resnick D. *Diagnosis of Bone and Joint Disorders*. 4th ed. Philadelphia: Saunders; 2002:1312.)

from carpal boss syndrome. Carpal boss syndrome has a slight male predominance and a peak incidence in the middle of the third decade of life. Trauma is often the common denominator in the development of carpal boss syndrome.

SIGNS AND SYMPTOMS

On physical examination, the carpal boss appears as a bony protuberance that can be seen more easily by having the patient flex the wrist (Fig. 9.5). The pain associated with this action can be reproduced by applying pressure to the soft tissue overlying the carpal boss. Patients with carpal boss syndrome demonstrate a positive hunchback sign; that is, the examiner can appreciate a bony prominence when palpating the carpal boss (see Fig. 9.2). Occasionally an inflamed bursa may overlie the bony excrudescence and may confuse the diagnosis as the normal hard consistency of the carpal boss may be masked by the

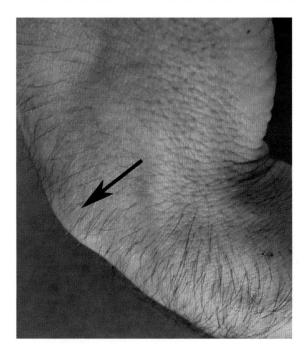

Fig. 9.5 With wrist flexion, the prominence of the carpal boss becomes strikingly evident *(arrow)*. (From Park MJ, Namdari S, Weiss A-P. The carpal boss: review of diagnosis and treatment. *J Hand Surg.* 2008;33(3):446–449 [Fig. 2]. ISSN 0363-5023, https://doi.org/10.1016/j.jhsa.2007.11.029, http://www.sciencedirect.com/science/article/pii/S0363502307011069.)

softer bursa. With acute trauma to the dorsum of the hand, ecchymosis over the carpal boss of the affected joint(s) may be present. Unlike the ganglion cysts of the wrist, which will transilluminate, the bony exostosis of the carpal boss will not transilluminate.

TESTING

Plain radiographs are indicated in all patients who present with a carpal boss to rule out fractures and to identify exostoses responsible for the symptoms (see Figs. 9.3 and 9.4). Based on the patient's clinical presentation, additional testing may be warranted to exclude inflammatory arthritis, including a complete blood count, erythrocyte sedimentation rate, uric acid level, and antinuclear antibody testing. Magnetic resonance imaging (MRI), computerized tomography (CT), and ultrasound imaging of the fingers and wrist are indicated if joint instability, occult mass, occult fracture, infection, or tumor is suspected, as well as to further assess the condition of the overlying tendons (Figs. 9.6 and 9.7). Radionuclide bone scanning may be useful to identify stress fractures (Fig. 9.8).

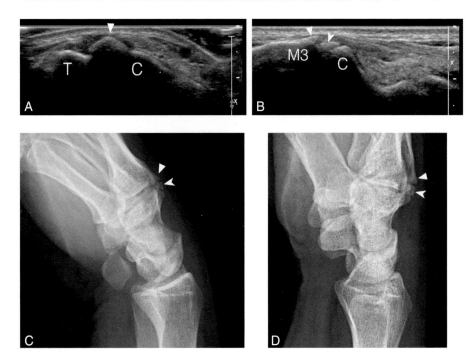

Fig. 9.6   A 36-year-old man with an asymptomatic palpable mass at the dorsal surface of his right wrist. Transverse (A) and longitudinal (B) ultrasound images obtained using a 12.5-MHz linear transducer on a Philips iu22 machine demonstrate a fragmented carpal boss at the dorsal base of the third metacarpal *(arrowheads)*, adjacent to the trapezoid *(T)* and capitate *(C)*. A radiograph from the same patient obtained with partial supination and ulnar deviation (C) improves conspicuity of the carpal boss *(arrowheads)* relative to the routine lateral view (D). (From Porrino J, Maloney E, Chew FS. Current concepts of the carpal boss: pathophysiology, symptoms, clinical or imaging diagnosis, and management. *Curr Prob Diag Radiol*. 2015;44(5):462–468 [Fig. 4]. ISSN 0363-0188, https://doi.org/10.1067/j.cpradiol.2015.02.008, http://www.sciencedirect.com/science/article/pii/S0363018815000274.)

DIFFERENTIAL DIAGNOSIS

The tentative diagnosis of carpal boss syndrome is made on clinical grounds and is confirmed by radiographic testing. Arthritis, tenosynovitis, or gout of the affected wrist may accompany carpal boss syndrome and exacerbate the patient's pain. Dorsal ganglion cysts may mimic the presentation of carpal boss. Occasionally an inflamed bursa may overlie the bony excrudescence and may confuse the diagnosis, as the normal hard consistency of the carpal boss may be masked by the softer bursa (Fig. 9.9). Occult fractures occasionally confuse the clinical presentation. Other pathologic processes that may mimic the clinical presentation of carpal boss include fibromas, osteomas, exuberant synovium, fracture callus, and a variety of tumors (Box 9.1).

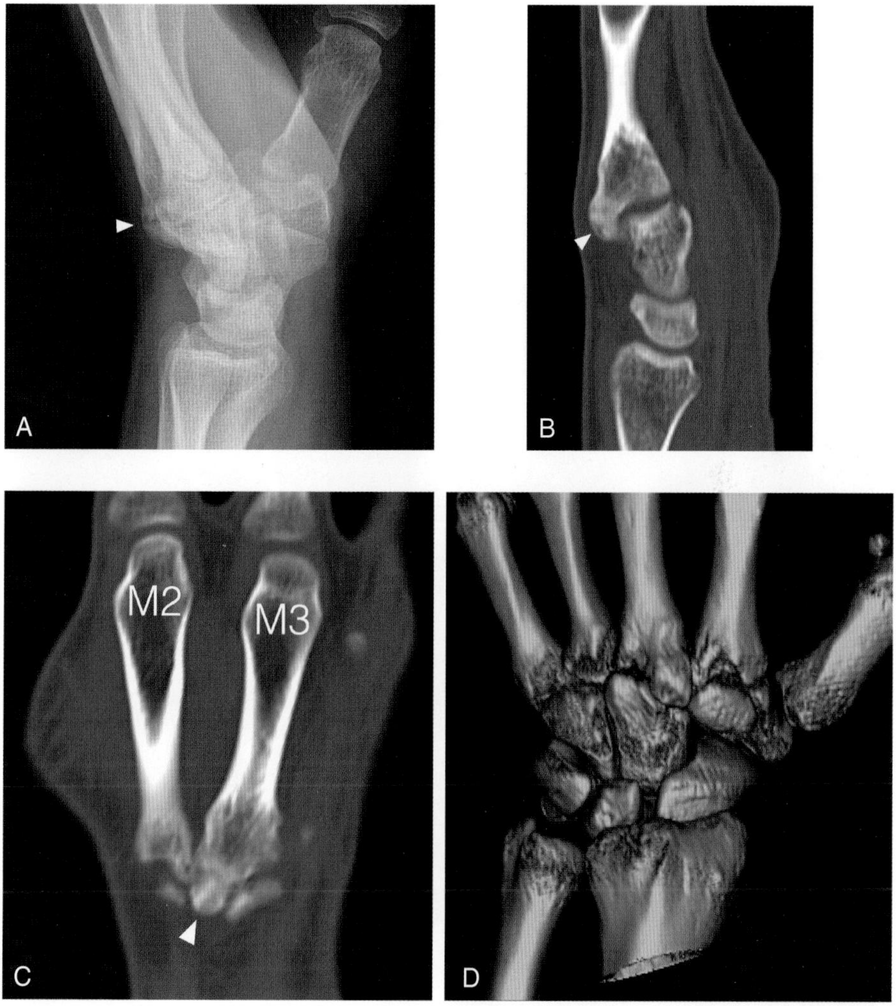

Fig. 9.7 A 28-year-old man with a palpable and painful mass at the dorsal surface of his left wrist. Lateral radiograph (A) demonstrates a carpal boss at the base of the third metacarpal *(arrowhead)*. Sagittal (B) and coronal (C) computed tomography images demonstrate an osseous protuberance emerging from the base of the third metacarpal and extending over the dorsal surface of the capitate and trapezoid, consistent with a carpal boss *(arrowheads)*. A three-dimensional reconstruction (D) demonstrates the carpal boss at the base of the third metacarpal, overlying the quadrangular trapezoid-capitate-metacarpal joint. *M2*, Second metacarpal; *M3*, third metacarpal. (From Porrino J, Maloney E, Chew FS. Current concepts of the carpal boss: pathophysiology, symptoms, clinical or imaging diagnosis, and management. *Curr Prob Diag Radiol.* 2015;44(5):462−468 [Fig. 5]. ISSN 0363-0188, https://doi.org/10.1067/j.cpradiol.2015.02.008, http://www.sciencedirect.com/science/article/pii/S0363018815000274.)

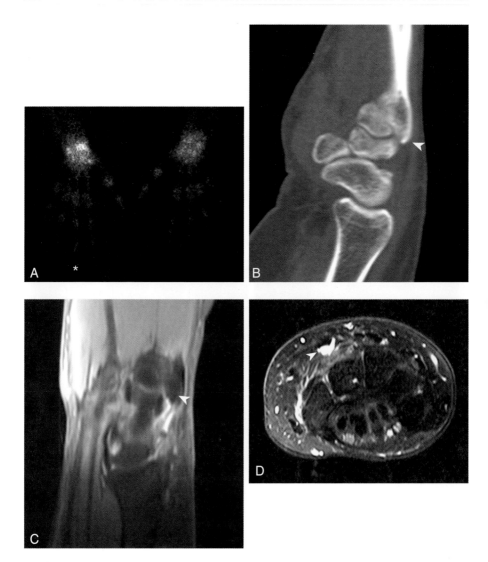

Fig. 9.8 A 39-year-old woman with dorsal wrist pain. Bone scan (A), acquired 3 hours after injection of 32mCi Tc-99m methyl diphosphonate, demonstrates increased radiotracer uptake in the left wrist *(asterisk)* compared with the right. Sagittal noncontrast computed tomography (B) and noncontrast proton-density fat-saturated magnetic resonance (MR) (C) images demonstrate a carpal boss at the base of the third metacarpal *(arrowhead)*. Noncontrast axial T2 fat-saturated MR image (D) just proximal to the carpal boss demonstrates abnormal fluid in the tendon sheath of the extensor carpi radialis brevis *(arrowhead)*, consistent with tenosynovitis. (From Porrino J, Maloney E, Chew FS. Current concepts of the carpal boss: pathophysiology, symptoms, clinical or imaging diagnosis, and management. *Curr Prob Diag Radiol.* 2015;44(5):462−468 [Fig. 2]. ISSN 0363-0188, https://doi.org/10.1067/j.cpradiol. 2015.02.008, http://www.sciencedirect.com/science/article/pii/S0363018815000274.)

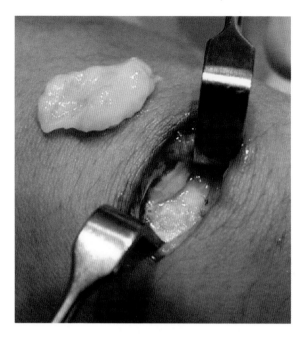

Fig. 9.9 Occasionally an inflamed bursa may overlie the bony excrudescence and may confuse the diagnosis, as the normal hard consistency of the carpal boss may be masked by the softer bursa. (From Park MJ, Namdari S, Weiss A-P. The carpal boss: review of diagnosis and treatment. *J Hand Surg.* 2008;33(3):446–449 [Fig. 4]. ISSN 0363-5023, https://doi.org/10.1016/j.jhsa.2007.11.029, http://www.sciencedirect.com/science/article/pii/S0363502307011069.)

BOX 9.1 ■ Differential Diagnosis of Carpal Boss

- Ganglion cyst
- Inflamed bursa
- Synovitis
- Fracture callus
- Exuberant synovium
- Fibroma
- Giant cell tumor
- Aneurysmal bone cyst
- Unicameral bone cyst
- Lipoma
- Neural tumors
- Interosseous ganglions
- Osteoid osteoma
- Osteochondroma
- Osteosarcoma
- Metastatic disease

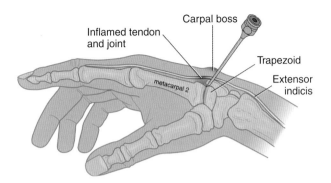

Fig. 9.10   Injection technique for carpal boss, or os styloideum. (From Waldman SD. Carpal boss. In: *Atlas of Pain Management Injection Techniques.* 2nd ed. Philadelphia: Saunders; 2007:268.)

TREATMENT

Initial treatment of the pain and functional disability associated with a carpal boss consists of nonsteroidal antiinflammatory drugs, simple analgesics, or cyclooxygenase-2 inhibitors. Physical modalities, including local heat and gentle range-of-motion exercises, should be introduced to avoid loss of function. Vigorous exercises should be avoided because they will exacerbate the patient's symptoms. A nighttime splint to protect the fingers may be helpful. If sleep disturbance is present, low-dose tricyclic antidepressants are indicated. If the patient does not respond to these conservative modalities, a trial of injection therapy with local anesthetic and steroid is a reasonable next step (Fig. 9.10). Rarely, surgical exploration and removal of the carpal boss are required for symptomatic relief.

HIGH-YIELD TAKEAWAYS

- The patient is afebrile, making an acute infectious etiology unlikely.
- The patient's symptomatology is most likely due to trauma to the wrist from a fall from a ladder.
- Physical examination and testing should be focused on the identification of the other pathologic processes that may mimic the clinical diagnosis of carpal boss.
- The patient exhibits the physical examination findings that are highly suggestive of carpal boss.
- The patient's symptoms are localized.
- Plain radiographs of the wrist will help identify bony abnormalities of the wrist, including fractures, dislocations, and osseous tumors.
- Ultrasound imaging, CT scanning, and MRI of the wrist and pelvis may help identify less common causes of wrist pain.

Suggested Readings

Alemohammad AM, Nakamura K, El-Sheneway M, Viegas SF. Incidence of carpal boss and osseous coalition: an anatomic study. *J Hand Surg Am.* 2009;34:1–6.

Capo JT, Orillaza NS, Lim PK. Carpal boss in an adolescent: case report. *J Hand Surg Am.* 2009;34:1808–1810.

Ghatan AC, Erik JC, Edward AA, Andrew JW. Attrition or rupture of digital extensor tendons due to carpal boss: report of 2 cases. *J Hand Surg.* 2014;39(5): 919–922.

Melone Jr. CP, Polatsch DB, Beldner S. Disabling hand injuries in boxing: boxer's knuckle and traumatic carpal boss. *Clin Sports Med.* 2009;28:609–621.

Park MJ, Namdari S, Weiss AP: The carpal boss: review of diagnosis and treatment. *J Hand Surg Am.* 2008;33:446–449.

Waldman SD. Carpal Boss. In: *Atlas of Common Pain Syndromes.* 4th ed. Philadelphia: Elsevier; 2019:231–235.

Karen Carpenter

A 19-Year-Old Female With Persistent Wrist Pain After Being Thrown From a Horse

LEARNING OBJECTIVES

- Learn the common causes of wrist pain.
- Develop an understanding of the unique vascular anatomy of the scaphoid bone.
- Develop an understanding of the causes of avascular necrosis of the scaphoid.
- Learn the clinical presentation of avascular necrosis of the scaphoid bone.
- Learn how to use physical examination to identify pathology of the scaphoid bone.
- Develop an understanding of the treatment options for avascular necrosis of the scaphoid bone.
- Learn the appropriate testing options to help diagnose avascular necrosis of the scaphoid bone.
- Learn to identify red flags in patients who present with wrist pain.
- Develop an understanding of the role in interventional pain management in the treatment of wrist pain.

Karen Carpenter

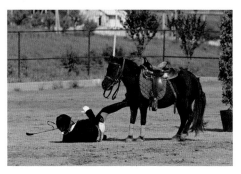 I entered the treatment room and sat down in front of my last patient and introduced myself. The young lady sitting in front of me stuck out her hand and said, "My name is Karen Carpenter. Not *that* Karen Carpenter, of course, but Karen Carpenter just the same." Her parents must have really liked "Close to You" or something. Well, it could be worse. "So, what brings you here today, Karen Carpenter?" I asked. "My wrist has been getting more painful ever since Bitsy threw me." "Bitsy?" I asked. "Oh, sorry, Bitsy is my horse. I love showing horses, and Bitsy is a real beauty. Gentle and very, very regal. I can't believe that she threw me! I have no idea what spooked her, but one minute we were prancing around the arena, and the next minute I was flying through the air. Good thing I had my helmet on, but right over her head I went. I landed right on my outstretched hand. You know, Doctor, I was so surprised, I didn't realize that I was hurt until an hour later when my right wrist really started hurting. I went to the ER, and they took x-rays and said nothing was broken, that it was just a strain, but I am 2 months out and it is getting harder and harder to hold my cell phone or type on my laptop. My friend Keely Donohoe recommended you. She said you fixed her knee up after her skiing accident last winter." I smiled and told her I was glad to hear that Keely was doing well.

I asked her what she had tried to help with the pain, and she said that she had tried rubbing on the Australian Dream, wore a wrist brace she got at the CVS, and took some Tylenol, but the pain just wasn't getting any better. Karen also noted that sometimes she used a heating pad, but she fell asleep with it on and she accidently burned herself.

I asked Karen if she had ever injured her wrist before. She thought for a moment, then said, "No. I broke my arm falling off the slide at the playground when I was little, but that was a long time ago." I asked Karen if she had ever taken any steroids, and she shook her head no and volunteered that the only medications she is on are her birth control pills.

I asked Karen to point with one finger to show me "where it hurts the most." She pointed to the base of her right thumb and said, "Doctor, it hurts way down deep, and it really gets my attention whenever I try to use my right hand." I asked, "Does the pain radiate anywhere?" Karen noted that sometimes it "ached down deep in the bone." Karen denied any gynecologic symptoms or blood in her urine.

On physical examination, Karen was afebrile and dyspneic at rest. Her respirations were 16. Her pulse was 88 and regular. Her blood pressure (BP) was normal at 112/76. Her head, eyes, ears, nose, throat (HEENT) exam was normal, as was her thyroid examination. Her cardiopulmonary examination was also normal. Her abdominal examination revealed no abnormal mass or organomegaly. There was no costovertebral angle (CVA) tenderness. There was no peripheral edema. Her low back examination was unremarkable. Visual inspection of the radial aspect of the right wrist revealed no cutaneous lesions or evidence of infection. There was no obvious bony deformity that would suggest a previous fracture. The area overlying the right scaphoid was cool to touch. Palpation of the area over the anatomic snuff box revealed mild diffuse tenderness, with no obvious effusion or point tenderness. There was mild crepitus, and I thought I detected a click with range of motion. The overall range of motion was decreased with pain exacerbated with active and passive range of motion, especially on radial deviation of the wrist. The Finkelstein test was negative bilaterally. The left wrist examination was normal, as was examination of her other major joints. A careful neurologic examination of the upper and lower extremities revealed there was no evidence of peripheral or entrapment neuropathy, and the deep tendon reflexes were normal.

Key Clinical Points—What's Important and What's Not

THE HISTORY

- A history of increasing right wrist pain after being thrown from a horse onto the outstretched hand
- No fractures of the wrist identified on x-ray at the time of the acute injury
- Increase in pain with use of the wrist
- No history of previous steroid use
- No history of previous trauma to the right wrist
- No fever or chills

THE PHYSICAL EXAMINATION

- Patient is afebrile
- Normal visual inspection of skin over the scaphoid
- Palpation of anatomic snuff box on the right reveals diffuse tenderness
- No point tenderness
- No increased temperature over the right scaphoid
- Crepitus to palpation during range of motion of right scaphoid
- Click sensation during range of motion of right scaphoid
- Negative Finkelstein test

OTHER FINDINGS OF NOTE

- Normal BP
- Normal HEENT examination
- Normal cardiovascular examination
- Normal pulmonary examination
- Normal abdominal examination
- No peripheral edema
- No groin mass or inguinal hernia
- No CVA tenderness
- Normal upper extremity neurologic examination, motor and sensory examination
- Examination of joints other than the right scaphoid were normal

What Tests Would You Like to Order?

The following tests were ordered:
- Plain radiograph of the right wrist with special attention to the scaphoid
- Magnetic resonance imaging (MRI) of the right wrist with special attention to the scaphoid

TEST RESULTS

The plain radiographs of the right scaphoid revealed an apparent cyst in the scaphoid but no fracture line (Fig. 10.1). The MRI of the right scaphoid confirms avascular necrosis in the proximal pole (Fig. 10.2).

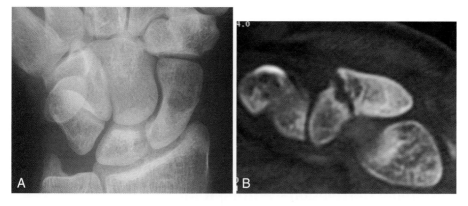

Fig. 10.1   (A) Radiograph obtained 12 weeks after a fall on an outstretched hand. There is an apparent cyst in the scaphoid but no fracture line. (B) Computed tomography scan, however, confirms fracture nonunion. (From Waldman S, Campbell R. *Imaging of Pain*. Philadelphia: Saunders; 2011 [Fig. 123-1].)

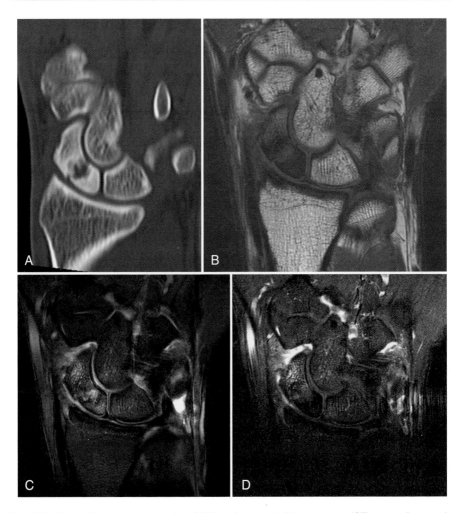

Fig. 10.2   Magnetic resonance imaging (MRI) and computed tomography (CT) scan of avascular necrosis (AVN) of the scaphoid. (A) CT scan of a patient with a scaphoid nonunion. The proximal pole is sclerotic, suggesting AVN. (B) T1-weighted (T1W) MRI shows low signal intensity (SI) of the proximal pole. (C, D) The lack of high SI enhancement on this postcontrast fat-saturated T1W MRI confirms AVN in the proximal pole. (From Waldman S, Campbell R. *Imaging of Pain*. Philadelphia: Saunders; 2011 [Fig. 123-3].)

Clinical Correlation—Putting It All Together

What is the diagnosis?

- Avascular necrosis (osteonecrosis) of the right scaphoid bone

The Science Behind the Diagnosis

ANATOMY OF THE BLOOD SUPPLY OF THE SCAPHOID BONE

Avascular necrosis of the scaphoid is a common sequela to scaphoid fracture. Second only to the hip in the incidence of avascular necrosis, the scaphoid is extremely susceptible to this disease because of the tenuous blood supply of the scaphoid, which enters the bone through its distal half. The dorsal blood supply and the volar blood supply are easily disrupted by fracture of the scaphoid, often leaving the proximal portion of the bone without nutrition due to loss of interosseous blood flow, leading to osteonecrosis (Fig. 10.3).

CLINICAL PRESENTATION

Common causes of scaphoid fracture include trauma to the scaphoid from falls on a hyperextended wrist, from prolonged high-dose steroid use, and from steering wheel injuries during motor vehicle accidents, although an idiopathic form of the disease, known as Preiser disease, can occur (Fig. 10.4; Box 10.1). A patient with avascular necrosis of the scaphoid will complain of deep unilateral wrist pain over the anatomic snuff box that may radiate into the radial aspect of the forearm and decreasing range of motion of the wrist. Weakened grip strength also may be noticed. Movement of the thumb usually exacerbates the patient's pain.

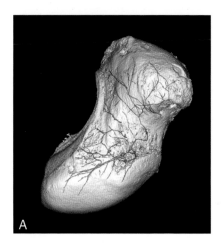
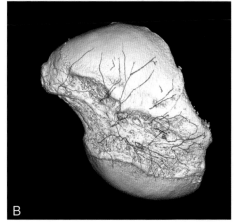

Fig. 10.3 Three-dimensional rendering of a scaphoid specimen with the intraosseous vasculature shows (A) the volar surface and (B) the lateral surface. (From Morsy M, Sabbagh MD, van Alphen NA, et al. The vascular anatomy of the scaphoid: new discoveries using micro—computed tomography imaging. *J Hand Surg.* 2019;44(11):928—938 [Fig. 1]. ISSN 0363-5023, https://doi.org/10.1016/j.jhsa.2019.08.001, http://www.sciencedirect.com/science/article/pii/S0363502318316393.)

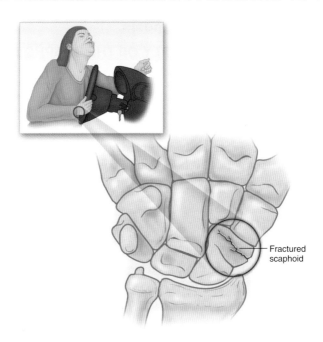

Fig. 10.4 Common causes of scaphoid fractures include trauma to the scaphoid from falls on a hyper-extended wrist and from steering wheel injuries during motor vehicle accidents. (From Waldman S. *Atlas of Uncommon Pain Syndromes*. 4th ed. Philadelphia: Elsevier; 2020 [Fig. 61-1].)

BOX 10.1 ■ Predisposing Factors for Avascular Necrosis of the Scaphoid

Trauma to wrist, especially falling on the outstretched hand
Corticosteroid use
Cushing disease
Alcohol abuse
Connective tissue diseases, especially systemic lupus erythematosus
Osteomyelitis
Human immunodeficiency virus
Organ transplantation
Hemoglobinopathies, including sickle cell disease
Hyperlipidemia
Gout
Renal failure
Pregnancy
Radiation therapy

SIGNS AND SYMPTOMS

Physical examination of patients suffering from avascular necrosis of the scaphoid will reveal pain on palpation of the anatomic snuff box (Fig. 10.5). The pain

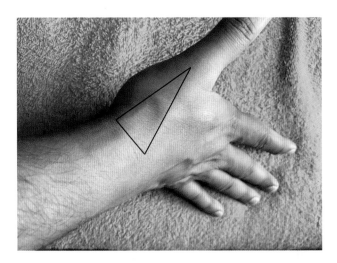

Fig. 10.5   Right hand in semi-prone position showing a triangular depression (anatomical snuff box) on the dorso-racial aspect. (From Deora S, Agrawal D, Choudhary R, Kaushik A, Patel T. Anatomical snuff box approach for percutaneous coronary interventions—current status. *Indian Heart Journal*. 2021;73(5): 539–543 [Fig 1].)

can be worsened by passively moving the wrist from ulnar to radial position or by moving the thumb of the affected side. A click or crepitus also may be appreciated by the examiner when putting the wrist through range of motion. Weakness of dorsiflexion is common, as is weakness of grip strength in contrast to the nonaffected side.

TESTING

Plain radiographs are indicated in all patients who present with avascular necrosis of the scaphoid to rule out underlying occult bony pathologic conditions and identify sclerosis and fragmentation of the scaphoid, although early in the course of the disease plain radiographs can be notoriously unreliable (Fig. 10.6). Based on the patient's clinical presentation, additional tests, including complete blood cell count, uric acid level, erythrocyte sedimentation rate, and antinuclear antibody testing, also may be indicated. Computerized tomography (CT) and MRI of the wrist are indicated in all patients thought to have avascular necrosis of the scaphoid or if other causes of joint instability, infection, or tumor are suspected (see Fig. 10.2). Administration of gadolinium followed by postcontrast imaging may help delineate the adequacy of blood supply, with contrast enhancement of the proximal scaphoid being a good prognostic sign (Fig. 10.7). Ultrasound imaging of the scaphoid also may aid in the diagnosis (Fig. 10.8). Electromyography is indicated if coexistent ulnar or carpal tunnel syndrome is suspected. A very gentle

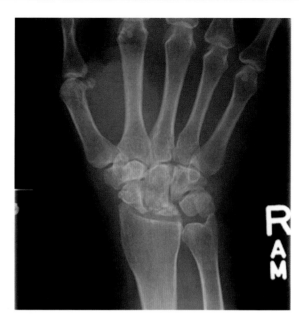

Fig. 10.6   Posteroanterior radiograph demonstrating avascular necrosis of the scaphoid and lunate. (From Budoff JE. Concomitant Kienböck's and Preiser's diseases: a case report. *J Hand Surg.* 2006;31(7): 1149–1153 [Fig. 1].)

injection of the radial aspect of the distal radioulnar joint with small volumes of local anesthetic and steroid provides immediate improvement of the pain, but ultimately surgical repair is required.

DIFFERENTIAL DIAGNOSIS

Coexistent arthritis and gout of the radioulnar, carpometacarpal, and interphalangeal joints; dorsal wrist ganglion; and tendinitis may occur with avascular necrosis of the scaphoid and exacerbate the patient's pain and disability. Distal fractures of the radius, de Quervain stenosis, tenosynovitis, scapholunate ligament tears, scaphoid cysts, contusions, and fractures also may mimic the pain of avascular necrosis of the scaphoid, as can tear of the triangular fibrocartilage complex (Box 10.2).

TREATMENT

Initial treatment of the pain and functional disability associated with avascular necrosis of the scaphoid should include a combination of nonsteroidal antiinflammatory drugs or cyclooxygenase-2 inhibitors and short-term immobilization of the wrist. Local application of heat and cold also may be beneficial. For

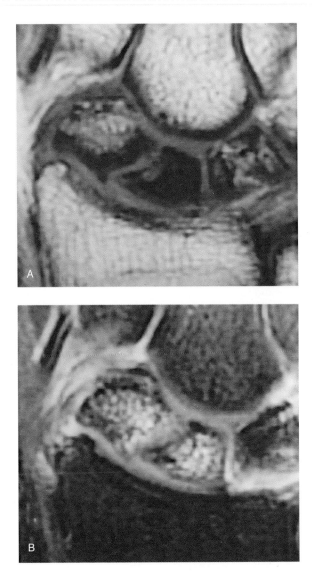

Fig. 10.7   Osteonecrosis of the scaphoid bone after a fracture. (A) Four months after a scaphoid fracture, coronal T1-weighted (TR/TE, 500/14) spin echo magnetic resonance imaging (MRI) reveals nonunion of the bone and low signal intensity at the fracture line and in the proximal pole of the scaphoid. (B) After intravenous gadolinium administration, fat-suppressed coronal T1-weighted (TR/TE, 550/14) spin echo MRI image shows enhancement in both portions of the scaphoid, a good prognostic sign. (From Resnick D, ed. *Diagnosis of Bone and Joint Disorders*. 4th ed. Philadelphia: Saunders; 2002:3045.)

patients who do not respond to these treatment modalities, gentle injection of a local anesthetic and steroid into the radial aspect of the distal radioulnar joint may be a reasonable next step to provide palliation of acute pain. Vigorous

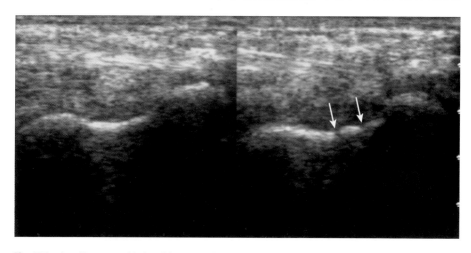

Fig. 10.8 A split-screen side-by-side comparison of the fractured scaphoid *(right)* and normal scaphoid *(left)*. The arrows identify two cortical fractures in the palmar cortex. (From Senall JA, Failla JM, Bouffard A, et al. Ultrasound for the early diagnosis of clinically suspected scaphoid fracture. *J Hand Surg Am.* 2004;29:400–405.)

BOX 10.2 ■ Differential Diagnosis for Avascular Necrosis of the Scaphoid

Scaphoid fracture
Scapholunate ligament tear
De Quervain stenosing tenosynovitis
Calcific tendinitis
Distal radius fracture
Distal radioulnar instability

---

exercises should be avoided because they exacerbate the patient's symptoms. Ultimately, surgical repair is the treatment of choice.

H I G H - Y I E L D   T A K E A W A Y S

- The patient is afebrile, making an acute infectious etiology (e.g., septic arthritis) unlikely.
- The patient's symptomatology is the result of acute trauma.
- The history of a fall onto the outstretched hand should raise the index of suspicion of avascular necrosis of the scaphoid.
- The patient's pain is diffuse and deeply aching rather than highly localized as would be the case in the sharp, severe, localized pain of de Quervain tenosynovitis.

(Continued)

- The patient's symptoms are unilateral and involve only one joint, which is more suggestive of a local process than a systemic polyarthropathy.
- Plain radiographs will provide high-yield information regarding the bony contents of the joint, but ultrasound imaging and MRI will be more useful in identifying soft tissue pathology.
- Bone scan may be useful in identifying fracture or avascular necrosis of the scaphoid not seen on x-ray.

Suggested Readings

Waldman SD. Avascular necrosis of the scaphoid. In: *Atlas of Uncommon Pain Syndromes*. 4th ed. Philadelphia: Elsevier; 2017:206—208.

Waldman SD. Intra-articular injection of the wrist joint. In: *Atlas of Pain Management Injection Techniques*. 4th ed. Philadelphia: Elsevier; 2017:250—253.

Waldman SD, Campbell RSD. Non-union of the scaphoid. In: *Imaging of Pain*. Philadelphia: Saunders; 2011:313—315.

Marco Arco

A 22-Year-Old Male With Severe Right Wrist Pain

- Learn the common causes of wrist pain.
- Develop an understanding of the unique anatomy of the wrist joint.
- Develop an understanding of the musculotendinous units that surround the wrist joint.
- Develop an understanding of the causes of flexor carpi ulnaris tendinitis.
- Develop an understanding of the differential diagnosis of flexor carpi ulnaris tendinitis.
- Learn the clinical presentation of flexor carpi ulnaris tendinitis.
- Learn how to examine the wrist.
- Learn how to use physical examination to identify flexor carpi ulnaris tendinitis.
- Develop an understanding of the treatment options for flexor carpi ulnaris tendinitis.

Marco Arco

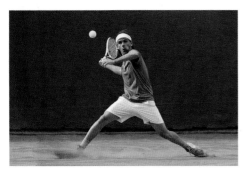

Marco Arco is a 22-year-old tennis player with the chief complaint of "I can't play tennis because my right wrist is killing me." Marco stated that he recently competed in a regional tennis tournament, and since then his right wrist has been extremely painful. "Doc, the competition was really tough, and the clay courts were not up to par. My game was really off that day. I was up against this guy from Spain in the semifinals, and we were really evenly matched. He sensed my backhand was not my strongest play, so he used it against me. The game went on for what seemed like hours, and neither of us could bring the game home. I was getting tired and so was he, but I felt like if I could hang on, I could win the thing. I started returning every ball as hard as I could. I knew it was a bad idea, but I just couldn't help myself. I wanted to win so bad! By match point, my right wrist was hurting so bad I could barely hold my racquet. I served one as hard as I could. I really put my whole body into that serve, and I knew there was no way that guy was going to return it. I won—he didn't—but from then on, the pinky finger side of my wrist has been really hurting. Especially in the mornings when I try to pick up my coffee mug. I feel a catch and a sharp pain."

I asked Marco about any antecedent wrist trauma, and he said he had strained his wrist several times in the past. "It always got better," he said, "but not this time." I asked what made the pain better, and he said that a couple of Aleves washed down with a Red Bull seemed to help. I asked Marco what made it worse, and he said the heating pad and anything that required him to move his wrist or lift anything with his right hand. I asked how he was sleeping, and he said, "Not worth a crap. I can't lay on my right side, and that's the side I like to sleep on. Every time I roll over, I get a sharp pain in the little finger side of my wrist and it wakes me up. I have a tough time getting back to sleep." He denied fever and chills. I asked Marco to point with one finger where it hurt the most. He pointed to the volar-ulnar aspect of the wrist just below the base of the little finger.

On physical examination, Marco was afebrile. His respirations were 16, and his pulse was 72 and regular. He was normotensive with a blood pressure of 120/70. Marco's head, eyes, ears, nose, throat (HEENT) exam was normal. His cardiopulmonary examination was normal. His thyroid was normal, as was his abdominal examination, which revealed no abnormal mass or organomegaly. There was no costovertebral angle (CVA) tenderness or peripheral edema.

Marco's low back examination was unremarkable. Visual inspection of the right wrist was normal, specifically there was no rubor. I noted that Marco was splinting his right wrist by holding it against his abdomen. The volar-ulnar aspect of the right wrist was a little warm, but it did not appear to be infected. There was marked point tenderness 2 to 3 cm above the pisiform. Active resisted ulnar deviation of the wrist as well as active resisted wrist flexion caused Marco to wince in pain. The left wrist examination was normal, as was examination of his other major joints. A careful neurologic examination of the upper extremities revealed there was no evidence of peripheral or entrapment neuropathy, and the deep tendon reflexes were normal.

Key Clinical Points—What's Important and What's Not

THE HISTORY

- A history of acute trauma following overuse of the wrist while playing tennis
- Previous history of wrist strains
- No fever or chills
- Acute onset of wrist pain with exacerbation of pain with wrist use
- Pain in the right wrist by the little finger
- Sleep disturbance
- Difficulty using wrist when lifting his coffee cup

THE PHYSICAL EXAMINATION

- Patient is afebrile
- Point tenderness to palpation of the volar-ulnar aspect of the wrist
- Palpation of volar-ulnar aspect of right wrist reveals warmth to touch
- A catching sensation and exacerbation of pain with active resisted adduction and flexion of the right wrist
- No evidence of infection

OTHER FINDINGS OF NOTE

- Normal HEENT examination
- Normal cardiovascular examination
- Normal pulmonary examination
- Normal abdominal examination
- No peripheral edema
- Normal upper extremity neurologic examination, motor and sensory examination
- Examinations of joints other than the right wrist were normal

What Tests Would You Like to Order?

The following tests were ordered:
- Plain radiographs of the right wrist
- Ultrasound of the right wrist

TEST RESULTS

The plain radiographs of the right wrist revealed a small area of calcification just proximal to the pisiform consistent with calcific tendinitis of the flexor carpi

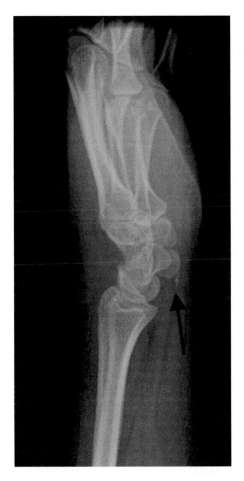

Fig. 11.1 Calcification is evident below the pisiform *(arrow)*, consistent with calcific tendinitis of the flexor carpi ulnaris tendon on this lateral radiograph of the hand. (From Steinbach LS. Calcium pyrophosphate dihydrate and calcium hydroxyapatite crystal deposition diseases: imaging perspectives. *Radiol Clin North Am.* 2004;42(1):185–205.)

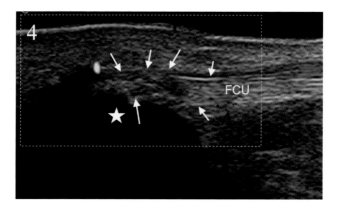

Fig. 11.2   Sagittal high-frequency ultrasound image of an active flexi carpi ulnaris (FCU) tendon entheso-pathy (i.e., the simultaneous sonomorphologic occurrence of tendon thickening and tendon hypo-echogenity with loss of the fibrillar echotexture [arrows], in a 45-year-old woman with painful pisiform overuse). The ★ indicates the pisiform. (From Wick MC, Weiss RJ, Arora R, et al. Enthesopathy of the flexor carpi ulnaris at the pisiform: Findings of high-frequency sonography. *Eur J Radiol.* 2011;77 (2):240–244.)

ulnaris (Fig. 11.1). Ultrasound examination of the right wrist revealed a thicken-ing and loss of the expected fibular echotexture of the flexor carpi ulnaris (Fig. 11.2).

 ## Clinical Correlation—Putting It All Together

What is the diagnosis?
- Flexor carpi ulnaris tendinitis

The Science Behind the Diagnosis
ANATOMY

Located in the forearm, the flexor carpi ulnaris muscle serves to flex and adduct (radially deviate) the hand (Fig. 11.3). The flexor carpi ulnaris muscle has two heads, which find their origin on the medial epicondyle of the humerus and the medial margin of the olecranon process of the ulna. The muscle finds its insertion on the pisiform bone with a secondary insertion via ligaments to the hamate, the third and fifth metacarpals, and the tuberosity of the trapezium (Figs. 11.4, 11.5 and 11.6). The flexor carpi ulnaris muscle is innervated by the median nerve and receives its blood supply from the ulnar artery. It is at its points of insertion and at the point at which the distal flexor carpi ulnaris musculotendinous unit passes beneath the flexor retinaculum that it is susceptible to the development of tendi-nitis, tears, and rupture (Fig. 11.7).

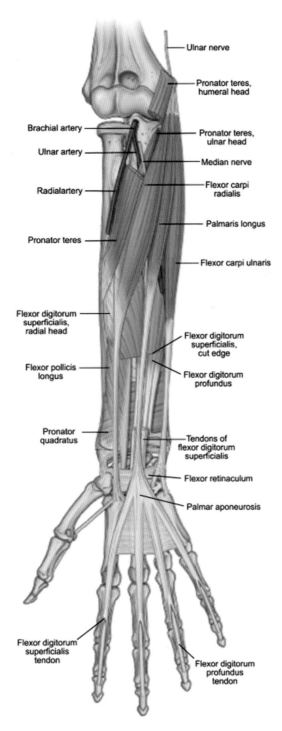

Fig. 11.3 The flexor capri ulnaris muscle. (From Wilson PD. *Anatomy of Muscle, Reference Module in Biomedical Sciences*. Elsevier; 2014 [Fig. 12]. ISBN 9780128012383, https://doi.org/10.1016/B978-0-12-801238-3.00250-6, http://www.sciencedirect.com/science/article/pii/B9780128012383002506.)

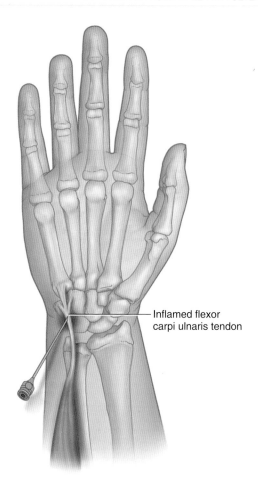

Inflamed flexor
carpi ulnaris tendon

Fig. 11.4 The flexor carpi ulnaris muscle finds its insertion on the pisiform bone with a secondary insertion via ligaments to the hamate, the third and fifth metacarpals, and the tuberosity of the trapezium. (From Waldman S. *Atlas of Pain Management Injection Techniques*. 4th ed. St. Louis: Elsevier; 2017 [Fig. 73-4].)

CLINICAL SYNDROME

The flexor carpi ulnaris tendon of the hand may develop tendinitis after overuse or misuse, especially when performing activities that require repeated flexion and adduction of the hand. Acute flexor carpi ulnaris tendinitis has been seen in clinical practice with increasing frequency owing to the increasing popularity of sports such as tennis, baseball, and golf (Fig. 11.8). Improper stretching of flexor carpi ulnaris muscle and flexor carpi ulnaris tendon before exercise has also been implicated in the development of flexor carpi ulnaris tendinitis, as well as acute tendon rupture. Injuries ranging from partial to complete tears of the tendon can

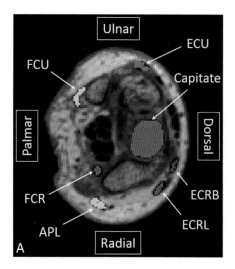
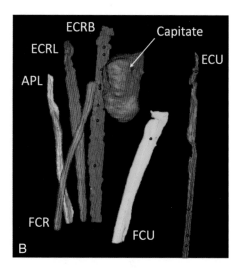

Fig. 11.5 The relationship of the various tendons of the wrist with the capitate as a point of orientation. (A) Cross section. (B) Coronal view. *APL*, Abductor pollicis longus; *ECRB*, extensor carpi radialis brevis; *ECRL*, extensor carpi radialis longus; *ECU*, extensor carpi ulnaris; *FCR*, flexor carpi radialis; *FCU*, flexor carpi ulnaris. (From Garland AK, Shah DS, Kedgley AE. Wrist tendon moment arms: quantification by imaging and experimental techniques. *J Biomech.* 2018;68:136–140 [Fig. 1]. ISSN 0021-9290, https://doi.org/10.1016/j.jbiomech.2017.12.024, http://www.sciencedirect.com/science/article/pii/S00219290173 07376.)

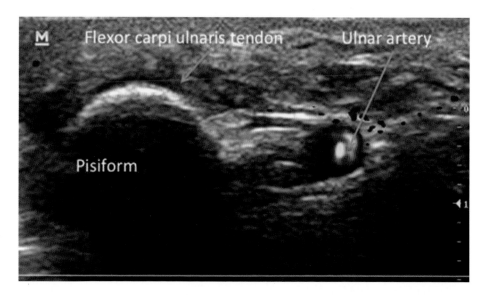

Fig. 11.6 Color Doppler ultrasound image demonstrating the flexor carpi ulnaris insertion on the pisaform. Note the relationship of the flexor carpi ulnaris tendon to the ulnar artery.

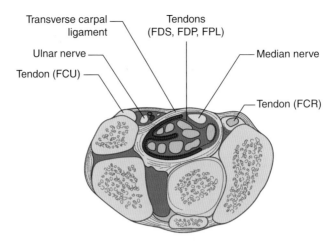

Fig. 11.7 The distal flexor carpi ulnaris musculotendious unit passes beneath the flexor retinaculum that it is susceptible to the development of tendinitis, tears, and rupture. *FCR*, flexor carpi radialis; *FCU*, flexor carpi ulnaris; *FdS*, flexor digitorum superficialis; *FPL*, flexor digitorum profundus; *FDP*, flexor digitorum longus. (From Preston DC, Shapiro BE. *Electromyography and Neuromuscular Disorders*. 3rd ed. New York: Elsevier; 2013: 267–288.)

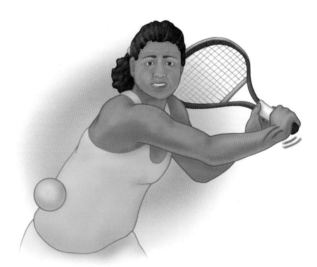

Fig. 11.8 The flexor carpi ulnaris tendon of the hand may develop tendinitis after overuse or misuse, especially when performing activities that require repeated flexion and adduction of the hand as when playing tennis, baseball, or racquetball. (From Waldman S. *Atlas of Common Pain Syndromes*. 4th ed. Philadelphia: Elsevier; 2019 [Fig. 51-1].)

occur when the distal tendon sustains direct trauma while it is fully flexed under load or when the wrist is forcibly flexed while the hand is in full radial deviation.

SIGNS AND SYMPTOMS

The pain of flexor carpi ulnaris tendinitis is constant and severe and is localized to the dorsoulnar aspect of the wrist. The patient suffering from flexor carpi ulnaris tendinitis often complains of sleep disturbance owing to pain. Patients with flexor carpi ulnaris tendinitis exhibit pain with active resisted flexion of the hand and with ulnar deviation of the wrist. In an effort to decrease pain, patients suffering from flexor carpi ulnaris tendinitis often splint the inflamed tendon by limiting hand flexion and ulnar deviation of the wrist to remove tension from the inflamed tendon. If untreated, patients suffering from flexor carpi ulnaris tendinitis may experience difficulty in performing any task that requires flexion and adduction of the wrist and hand, such as using a hammer or lifting a heavy coffee mug. Over time, if the tendinitis is not treated, muscle atrophy and calcific tendinitis may result, or the distal musculotendinous unit may suddenly rupture. Patients who experience complete rupture of the flexor carpi ulnaris tendon will not be able to fully and forcefully flex the hand or fully adduct the wrist.

TESTING

Plain radiographs are indicated in all patients who present with wrist and hand pain. Patients with flexor carpi ulnaris tendinitis will exhibit a characteristic fluffy calcification just above the tendon's insertion on the pisiform (Fig. 11.9). Based on the patient's clinical presentation, additional testing may be indicated, including complete blood cell count, sedimentation rate, and antinuclear antibody testing. Magnetic resonance imaging (MRI) or ultrasound imaging of the wrist and hand is indicated if flexor carpi ulnaris tendinopathy or tear is suspected. MRI or ultrasound evaluation of the affected area may also help delineate the presence of calcific tendinitis or other hand pathology (Fig. 11.10; see also Fig. 11.2).

DIFFERENTIAL DIAGNOSIS

The differential diagnosis of ulnar-sided wrist pain should include extensor carpi ulnaris tendonitis, flexor carpi ulnaris tendonitis, pisotriquetral arthritis, triangular fibrocartilage complex lesions, ulnar impaction, lunotriquetral instability, hook of the hamate fracture, hypothenar hammer syndrome, and distal radioulnar joint instability (Box 11.1). Flexor carpi ulnaris is localized to the dorsoulnar aspect of the wrist and will worsen with flexion, distinguishing it from extensor carpi ulnaris tendonitis.

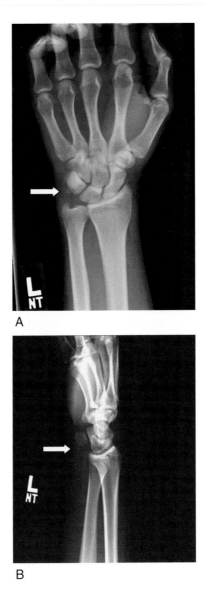

Fig. 11.9 Anteroposterior (A) and oblique (B) radiographs demonstrate a small area of calcification *(arrow)* just proxymal to the pisiform. (From Torbati SS, Bral D, Geiderman JM. Acute calcific tendinitis of the wrist. *J Emerg Med.* 2013;44(2):352—354 [Fig. 1].)

TREATMENT

Initial treatment of the pain and functional disability associated with flexor carpi ulnaris tendinitis includes a combination of nonsteroidal antiinflammatory drugs or cyclooxygenase-2 inhibitors and physical therapy. Local application of

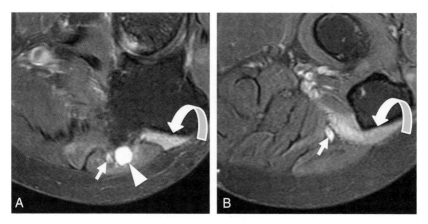

Fig. 11.10   Axial T2-weighted fat-saturated images at proximal forearm demonstrate an extraneural ganglion cyst arising from the ulnotrochlear margin of the joint (A, *arrowhead*). The cyst compresses the T2-weighted hyperintense and enlarged ulnar nerve (A, B, *arrows*) against the adjacent flexor carpi ulnaris. Denervation change is present in the proximal flexor digitorum profundus muscle (A, B, *curved arrows*). (From Howe BM, Spinner RJ, Felmlee JP, Frick MA. MR imaging of the nerves of the upper extremity: Elbow to wrist. *Magn Reson Imaging Clin N Am*. 2015;23(3):469–478.)

BOX 11.1 ■ Common Causes of Ulnar-Sided Wrist Pain

- Extensor carpi ulnaris tendonitis
- Flexor carpi ulnaris tendonitis
- Pisotriquetral arthritis
- Triangular fibrocartilage complex lesions
- Ulnar impaction
- Lunotriquetral instability
- Hook of the hamate fracture
- Hypothenar hammer syndrome
- Distal radioulnar joint instability

---

heat and cold may also be beneficial. Any repetitive activity that may exacerbate the patient's symptoms should be avoided. For patients who do not respond to these treatment modalities, injection of local anesthetic and steroid is a reasonable next step (see Fig. 11.4).

HIGH-YIELD TAKEAWAYS

- The patient is afebrile, making an acute infectious etiology (e.g., septic arthritis) unlikely.
- The patient's symptomatology is the result of acute overuse of the wrist, and physical examination and testing should be focused on the identification of

(Continued)

ligamentous injury, tendinitis, acute arthritis, and bursitis that may also be contributing to the patient's pain and functional disability.

• The patient has point tenderness over the insertion of the flexor carpi ulnaris tendon, which is highly suggestive of flexor carpi ulnaris tendinitis.

• There is warmth over the affected area suggestive of an inflammatory process.

• The patient's symptoms are unilateral and involve only one joint, which is more suggestive of a local process than a systemic polyarthropathy.

• Sleep disturbance is common and must be addressed concurrently with the patient's pain symptomatology.

• Plain radiographs will provide high-yield information regarding the bony contents of the joint, but ultrasound imaging and MRI will be more useful in identifying soft tissue pathology.

Suggested Readings

Fedorczyk JM. Tendinopathies of the elbow, wrist, and hand: histopathology and clinical considerations. *J Hand Ther*. 2012;25(2):191−201.

Henderson CJ, Kobayashi KM. Ulnar-sided wrist pain in the athlete. *Orthop Clin North Am*. 2016;47(4):789−798.

Patrick NC, Hammert WC. Hand and wrist tendinopathies. *Clin Sport Med*. 2020;39(2): 247−258.

Pirolo JM, Yao J. Minimally invasive approaches to ulnar-sided wrist disorders. *Hand Clin*. 2014;30(1):77−89.

Torbati SS, Bral D, Geiderman JM. Acute calcific tendinitis of the wrist. *J Emerg Med*. 2013;44(2):352−354.

Waldman SD. Flexor carpi ulnaris tendinitis. In: Waldman SD, ed. *Atlas of Common Pain Syndromes*. 4th ed. Elsevier; 2019:200−203.

Waldman SD. Flexor carpi ulnaris tendinitis and other disorders of the flexor carpi ulnaris. In: *Waldman's Comprehensive Atlas of Diagnostic Ultrasound of Painful Conditions*. Philadelphia: Wolters Kluwer; 2016:413−416.

Waldman SD. Flexor carpi ulnaris tendon injection. In: *Atlas of Pain Management Injection Techniques*. 4th ed. Philadelphia: Saunders; 2017:262−264.

Waldman SD. The biceps tendon. In: *Pain Review*. 2nd ed. Philadelphia: Elsevier; 2017: 91−92.

Waldman SD, Campbell RSD. Biceps tendinopathy. In: *Imaging of Pain*. Philadelphia: Saunders; 2011:245−246.

Birger Jakobsen

A 64-Year-Old Male With a Deformity of the Left Hand

- Learn the common causes of hand pain.
- Learn the common causes of hand deformity.
- Develop an understanding of the unique anatomy of the palmar fascia.
- Develop an understanding of the differential diagnosis of Dupuytren contracture.
- Learn to identify the underlying diseases associated with Dupuytren contracture.
- Learn the clinical presentation of Dupuytren contracture.
- Learn how to examine the hand to identify Dupuytren contracture.
- Learn how to use physical examination to identify Dupuytren contracture.
- Develop an understanding of the treatment options for Dupuytren contracture.

Birger Jakobsen

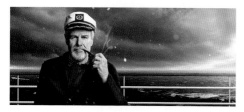

"You know, Doctor, my dad and older brother had this same thing," said *The Captain*. Everybody in my office called him *The Captain*. He had that command presence vibe: all seriousness and business. "I thought I might not get it, but just about the time I turned 60, I started getting these calluses on my palm. They hurt when I try to grab anything with my hand. I guess I didn't dodge the bullet. Like father, like son." Birger Jakobsen was a long-standing patient of the practice. He is a 64-year-old sea captain with the chief complaint of "I can't put on my gloves because my fingers won't straighten out." *The Captain* stated that over the last year, the calluses had turned into "bands that were tight as a hawser," and now he found it harder and harder to straighten out his fingers. He noted that as the fingers got more bent, the pain seemed to gradually get better. He noted that the pain was worse at night after a full day at work. He tried using a heating pad and Extra-Strength Tylenol without much success. *The Captain* noted, "Doctor, I worry that my hand could cause one of my crew to get hurt because my hand just doesn't work like it should. I really can't hold a fire extinguisher, and a fire at sea is my biggest fear." I could see that *The Captain* was really worried, and I tried to reassure him that we had some new treatments that weren't around when his dad was struggling with it.

The Captain denied any antecedent hand trauma. I asked what made the pain better, and he said, "Nothing really helps, but it's not about the pain." It was about his hand deformity. I asked Birger what made his pain worse, and he said, "Any time I have to use my hand. Like just about everything to do with my job!" Birger denied fever and chills, but reminded me that his "blood pressure was up and I take that blood pressure pill every day. So, Doctor, I am only *The Captain* to my crew, please just call me Birger. I was named after my grandpa, a real tough cookie, a proud Dane. I don't think I ever saw him smile." I smiled and said, "Okay, Birger it is. Let's take a look at that hand."

On physical examination, Birger was afebrile. His respirations were 18, and his pulse was 74 and regular. He was normotensive with a blood pressure of 126/74. His head, eyes, ears, nose, throat (HEENT) exam was normal, as was his cardiopulmonary examination. His thyroid was normal. His abdominal examination revealed no abnormal mass or organomegaly. There was no costovertebral angle (CVA) tenderness or peripheral edema. Birger's low back examination was unremarkable. Visual inspection of the right hand revealed findings with the later stages of Dupuytren contracture. He had the classic findings of

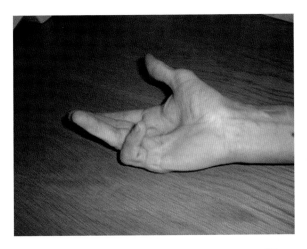

Fig. 12.1 This clinical photograph demonstrates the classic presentation of Dupuytren disease. The ulnar fingers show flexion contractures. (From Birks M, Bhalla A. Dupuytren's disease. *Surgery* (Oxford). 2013;31(4):177–180.)

Dupuytren: the dense, scarlike palmar contracture with a severe contraction of the little finger (Fig. 12.1). There was no rubor or color of the right hand, but there was diffuse tenderness to deep palpation of the fibrous cords. Range of motion of the right hand was limited, and his little finger was completely ankylosed. The left hand examination was normal, as was examination of his other major joints. A careful neurologic examination of the upper extremities revealed there was no evidence of peripheral or entrapment neuropathy, and the deep tendon reflexes were normal.

Key Clinical Points—What's Important and What's Not

THE HISTORY

- History of gradual onset of right hand pain and associated deformity
- Strong family history of similar right hand pain and deformity
- Patient of Danish descent
- History of gradual increase in deformity of the right hand
- History of gradual decrease in pain as the deformity worsened
- Inability to don gloves
- History of hypertension
- No history of previous significant hand pain
- No fever or chills
- Exacerbation of pain with hand use

- Increasing inability to carry out activities of daily living due to severe limitation of hand range of motion

THE PHYSICAL EXAMINATION

- Patient is afebrile
- Fibrous scar palmar contractures are present (see Fig. 12.1)
- Significant flexion contraction of the little finger on the right (see Fig. 12.1)
- No evidence of infection
- Pain on range of motion of the fingers of the right hand
- Extremely limited ability to fully extend the fingers of the right hand

OTHER FINDINGS OF NOTE

- Normal HEENT examination
- Normal cardiovascular examination
- Normal pulmonary examination
- Normal abdominal examination
- No peripheral edema
- Normal upper extremity neurologic examination, motor and sensory examination
- Examination of joints other than the right hand is normal

 ## What Tests Would You Like to Order?

The following tests were ordered:
- Plain radiographs of the right hand
- Ultrasound of the right hand

TEST RESULTS

The plain radiographs of the right hand revealed flexion deformities of the metacarpophalangeal joints and a severe flexion contracture of the fifth finger (Fig. 12.2). Ultrasound examination of the right hand revealed a large palmar fibromatosis consistent with a clinical diagnosis of Dupuytren disease (Fig. 12.3).

 ## Clinical Correlation—Putting It All Together

What is the diagnosis?
- Dupuytren contracture; Dupuytren disease

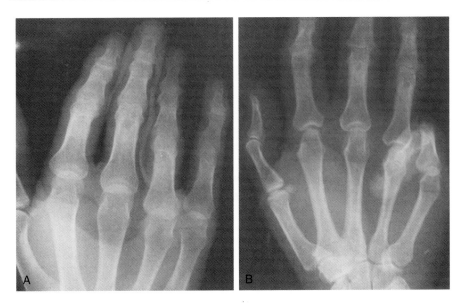

Fig. 12.2 Radiographic manifestations of Dupuytren contracture. (A) Flexion deformities of the meta-carpophalangeal joints of the four ulnar digits are demonstrated. (B) Severe flexion contracture is evident in the fifth finger, with minor changes in the other digits. (From Resnick D. *Diagnosis of Bone and Joint Disorders*, 4th ed. Philadelphia: Saunders; 2002:4667.)

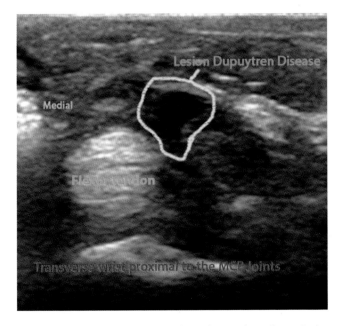

Fig. 12.3 Transverse ultrasound image demonstrating a large palmar fibromatosis associated with Dupuytren disease. (From Waldman S. *Atlas of Common Pain Syndromes*. 4th ed. Philadelphia: Elsevier; 2019 [Fig. 60-4].)

The Science Behind the Diagnosis

ANATOMY

Dupuytren contracture is the result of the thickening of the palmar fascia and its effect on the flexor tendons (Fig. 12.4). The primary function of the palmar fascia is to provide firm support to the overlying skin to aid the hand in gripping and to protect the underlying tendons.

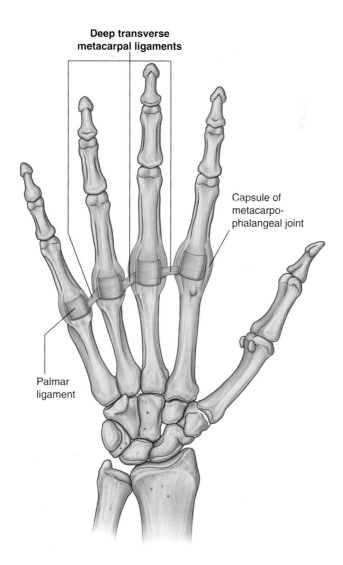

Fig. 12.4 The anatomy of the palmar fascia (aponeurosis). (From Drake R, Vogl W, Mitchell A. *Gray's Anatomy for Students*. 4th ed. Philadelphia: Churchill Livingstone; 2020 [Fig. 7.95].)

CLINICAL SYNDROME

Dupuytren contracture is a common complaint. Although it is initially painful, the pain seems to decrease as the condition progresses. As a result, patients suffering from Dupuytren contracture generally seek medical attention for functional disability rather than for pain.

Dupuytren contracture is caused by progressive fibrosis of the palmar fascia. Initially, the patient may notice fibrotic nodules along the course of the flexor tendons of the hand that are tender to palpation. As the disease advances, these nodules coalesce and form fibrous bands that gradually thicken and contract around the flexor tendons; this has the effect of drawing the affected fingers into flexion. Although any finger can develop Dupuytren contracture, the ring and little fingers are most commonly affected (Fig. 12.5). If untreated, the fingers can develop permanent flexion contractures. The plantar fascia may be affected concurrently.

Dupuytren contracture is thought to have a genetic basis and occurs most frequently in male patients of northern Scandinavian descent. It has an autosomal dominant inheritance pattern with variable penetrance. Siblings of patients suffering from Dupuytren contracture have three times the risk of developing the disease than the general population. Recent research has demonstrated that there are nine susceptibility loci with the strongest association with the clinical expression of the Dupuytren contracture located on an intron of *EPDR1*, the gene responsible for encoding the ependymin-related-1 protein. The disease may also be associated with trauma to the palm, diabetes, alcoholism, anticonvulsants, human immunodeficiency virus (HIV), and long-term barbiturate use. It is also believed that patients with Dupuytren disease are at increased risk of nonmelanoma skin cancer and psoriasis. Dupuytren disease rarely occurs before the fourth decade.

SIGNS AND SYMPTOMS

In the early stages of the disease, hard fibrotic nodules known as Garrod pads along the path of the flexor tendons can be palpated. These nodules are often misdiagnosed as calluses or warts (Fig. 12.6; Box 12.1). At this early stage, pain is invariably present. As the disease progresses, taut fibrous bands form; they may cross the metacarpophalangeal joint and ultimately the proximal interphalangeal joint (Fig. 12.7). These bands are not painful to palpation, and although they limit finger extension, finger flexion remains relatively normal. At this point, patients often seek medical advice because of difficulty putting on gloves and reaching into pockets. In the final stages of the disease, flexion contracture develops, with its negative impact on function (Fig. 12.8). Arthritis, gout of the metacarpal and interphalangeal joints, and trigger finger may coexist with Dupuytren contracture and may exacerbate the patient's pain and disability.

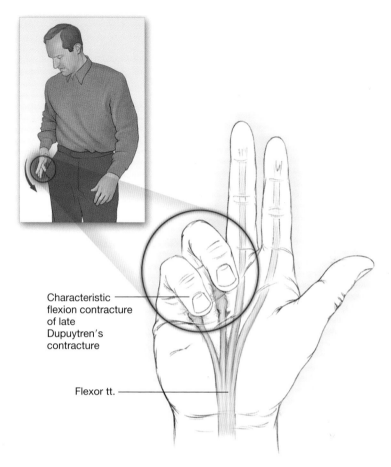

Characteristic
flexion contracture
of late
Dupuytren's
contracture

Flexor tt.

Fig. 12.5 Dupuytren contracture usually affects the fourth and fifth digits in men primarily of Scandinavian decent who are older than 40 years of age. (From Waldman S. *Atlas of Common Pain Syndromes*. 4th ed. Philadelphia: Elsevier; 2019 [Fig. 60-1].)

TESTING

Plain radiographs are indicated for all patients who present with Dupuytren contracture to rule out occult bony disease (see Fig. 12.2). Based on the patient's clinical presentation, additional testing may be warranted, including a complete blood count, uric acid level, erythrocyte sedimentation rate, and antinuclear antibody testing. Magnetic resonance imaging (MRI) and ultrasound imaging of the hand are indicated if joint instability or tumor is suspected, as well as to further evaluate the extent of the disease prior to surgical treatment (Figs. 12.9 and 12.10; see also Fig. 12.3). Electromyography is indicated if coexistent ulnar or carpal tunnel syndrome is a possibility.

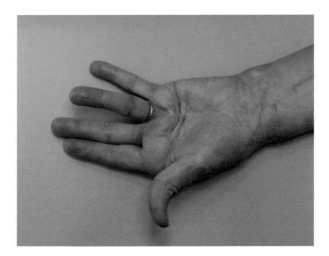

Fig. 12.6   Stage 1 of Dupuytren contracture presents as band in the palmar aponeurosis with skin tethering, puckering, and pitting. (From Bogdanov I, Payne CR. Dupuytren contracture as a sign of systemic disease. *Clin Dermatol.* 2019;37(6):675–678 [Fig. 1]. ISSN 0738-081X, https://doi.org/10.1016/j.clindermatol.2019.07.027, http://www.sciencedirect.com/science/article/pii/S0738081X19301385.)

BOX 12.1 ■ **Grading Classification of Dupuytren Disease**

- Grade 1: Presents as band in the palmar aponeurosis with skin tethering, puckering, and pitting
- Grade 2: Presents as a peritendinous band, and extension of the affected finger is limited
- Grade 3: Presents as a flexion contracture

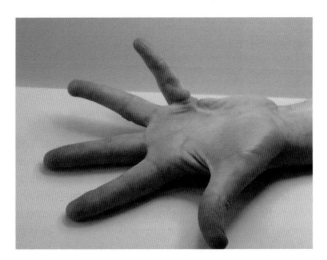

Fig. 12.7   Stage 2 presents as a peritendinous band, and extension of the affected finger is limited. (From Bogdanov I, Payne CR. Dupuytren contracture as a sign of systemic disease. *Clin Dermatol.* 2019;37(6):675–678 [Fig. 2]. ISSN 0738-081X, https://doi.org/10.1016/j.clindermatol.2019.07.027, http://www.sciencedirect.com/science/article/pii/S0738081X19301385.)

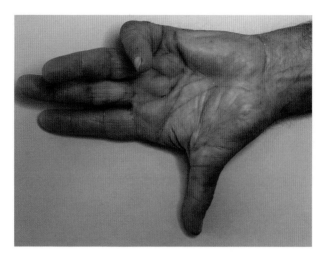

Fig. 12.8 Stage 3 of Dupuytren contracture presents as flexion contracture of the fifth digit. (From Bogdanov I, Payne CR. Dupuytren contracture as a sign of systemic disease. *Clin Dermatol*. 2019;37(6): 675–678 [Fig. 3]. ISSN 0738-081X, https://doi.org/10.1016/j.clindermatol.2019.07.027, http://www .sciencedirect.com/science/article/pii/S0738081X19301385.)

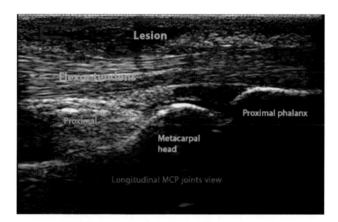

Fig. 12.9 Longitudinal ultrasound image demonstrating stage 1 Dupuytren contracture (palmar fibromatosis). Rounded hypoechoic solid fibroma *(arrows)* on the palmar aspect of the flexor tendon is the earliest sign of Dupuytren contracture of the hand. A plantar fibroma of the foot would be intimately related to the plantar fascia and have a similar appearance on ultrasound.

DIFFERENTIAL DIAGNOSIS

Dupuytren contracture is a clinically distinct entity that is rarely misdiagnosed once the syndrome is well established. Rarely, trigger finger or the claw hand associated with ulnar nerve pathology is misdiagnosed as Dupuytren contracture. Coexisting flexor tendinitis or trigger finger may be confused with Dupuytren

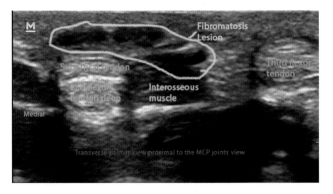

Fig 12.10 Transverse ultrasound image demonstrating the characteristic palmar fibromatosis associated with Dupuytren disease.

BOX 12.2 ■ Diseases That May Mimic Dupuytren Disease

- Ganglion cysts
- Callus formation
- Hyperkeratosis
- Rheumatoid nodules
- Palmar fibromatosis
- Pigmented villonodular synovitis
- Giant cell tumors
- Epithelioid sarcomas

---

contracture early in the course of the disease. Other diseases that may be confused for Dupuytren contracture include rheumatoid nodules, callus formation, hyperkeratosis, palmar fibromatosis, fibromas, and giant cell tumors (Box 12.2).

TREATMENT

Initial treatment of the pain and functional disability associated with Dupuytren contracture includes a combination of nonsteroidal antiinflammatory drugs or cyclooxygenase-2 inhibitors and physical therapy. A nighttime splint to protect the fingers may be helpful. If greater symptomatic relief is required, the injection of the fibrous scar contractures should be considered (Fig. 12.11).

Ultrasound needle guidance may improve the accuracy of needle placement. This technique can be used for the injection of collagenase *Clostridium histolyticum*, which is rapidly gaining acceptance as a nonsurgical treatment for Dupuytren contracture.

Physical modalities, including local heat and gentle range-of-motion exercises, should be introduced several days after the patient undergoes injection. Vigorous exercises should be avoided because they will exacerbate the patient's symptoms.

Although the foregoing treatment modalities provide symptomatic relief, Dupuytren contracture usually requires surgical treatment.

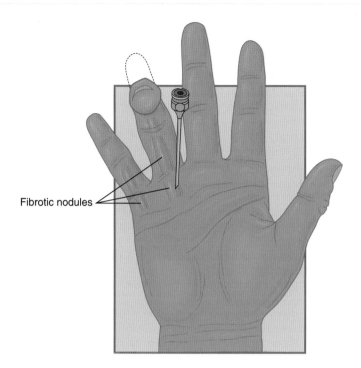

Fibrotic nodules

Fig. 12.11 Injection technique for the treatment of Dupuytren contracture. (From Waldman S. *Atlas of Pain Management Injection Techniques*. 4th ed. St. Louis: Elsevier; 2017 [Fig. 91-4].)

HIGH-YIELD TAKEAWAYS

- The patient is afebrile, making an acute infectious etiology (e.g., septic arthritis) unlikely.
- The diagnosis of Dupuytren contracture can usually be made on clinical grounds.
- It is seen more frequently in men and individuals of Scandinavian decent.
- The course of the disease is predictable with pain improving as the hand deformity worsens.
- The patient's symptomatology is significant, and physical examination and testing should be focused on the identification of other underlying treatable conditions known to be associated with Dupuytren contracture.
- The patient has significant negative impact on the ability to carry out activities of daily living and safely perform the job as a tanker captain.
- The patient's symptoms are unilateral and involve only one joint, which is more suggestive of a local process than a systemic polyarthropathy.
- Plain radiographs will provide high-yield information regarding the bony contents of the affected fingers, but arthrography, ultrasound imaging, and MRI will be more useful in identifying occult soft tissue pathology and confirming the extent of disease when planning surgical treatment.

Suggested Readings

Bogdanov I, Payne CR. Dupuytren contracture as a sign of systemic disease. *Clin Dermatol*. 2019;37(6):675–678.

Dutta A, Jayasinghe G, Deore S, et al. Dupuytren's contracture – current concepts. *J Clin Orthop Trauma*. 2020;11(4):590–596.

Fei TT, Chernoff E, Monacco NA, et al. Collagenase *Clostridium histolyticum* for the treatment of distal interphalangeal joint contractures in Dupuytren disease. *J Hand Surg*. 2019;44(5):417.e1–417.e4.

Kadhum M, Smock E, Khan A, et al. Radiotherapy in Dupuytren's disease: a systematic review of the evidence. *J Hand Surg (Eur Vol)*. 2017;42(7):689–692.

Mella JR, Guo L, Hung V. Dupuytren's contracture: an evidence-based review. *Ann Plast Surg*. 2018;81(6):S97–S101.

Nordenskjöld J, Englund M, Zhou C, et al. Prevalence and incidence of doctor-diagnosed Dupuytren's disease: a population-based study. *J Hand Surg (Eur Vol)*. 2017;42(7):673–677.

Waldman SD. Dupuytren's contracture. In: *Atlas of Common Pain Syndromes*. 4th ed. Philadelphia: Elsevier; 2019:236–238.

Waldman SD. Dupuytren's contracture. In: *Pain Review*. 2nd ed. Philadelphia: Elsevier; 2017:263–264.

Waldman SD. Dupuytren contracture injection. In: *Atlas of Pain Management Injection Techniques*. 4th ed. Philadelphia: Saunders; 2017:325–327.

Zhang D, Earp BE, Blazar P. Risk factors for skin tearing in collagenase treatment of Dupuytren contractures. *J Hand Surg*. 2019;44(12):1021–1025.

Jimmie "Guitar" Watson

A 27-Year-Old Male With a Finger That Locks Up When He Plays Guitar

- Learn the common causes of trigger finger.
- Develop an understanding of the unique anatomy of the flexor apparatus of the finger.
- Develop an understanding of the causes of trigger finger.
- Develop an understanding of the differential diagnosis of trigger finger.
- Learn the clinical presentation of trigger finger.
- Learn how to examine the finger and associated tendons.
- Learn how to use physical examination to identify trigger finger.
- Develop an understanding of the treatment options for trigger finger.

Jimmie "Guitar" Watson

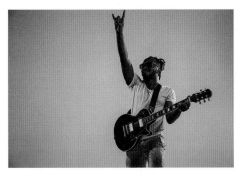

Jimmie "Guitar" Watson is a 27-year-old guitar player with the chief complaint of "the little finger on my left hand keeps locking up when I'm playing my guitar." Jimmie stated that ever since his band went on tour last fall, the middle finger on his left hand had been locking up. "Doc, the tour was amazing! We were the opening act for the $99^1/_2$ Blues band. We played an hour set to get the audience warmed up, and then we played backup for $99^1/_2$. We were playing 7 days a week straight for the entire 14-week tour. It was amazing! About the finger, first it would only lock up at the end of the evening, but as the tour was winding down, the finger would lock up all the time. I figured out some workarounds. I came up with a technique that avoids using the middle finger. I focus on using my thumb, index, and ring finger, with my pinky picking up the slack. Barring chords is off the table for now. I switched from my chunky neck Strat from the mid-60s to a '50s reissue that I found in a pawn shop in Little Rock. It has a soft V neck that is a little easier on the hand. Doctor, this finger locking up is really driving me crazy, though. At first it was just once in a while and sometimes it would straighten out on its own. But now once my finger locks, I have to stop strumming and reach up to straighten it out. I am afraid that one of these times it's going to lock up for good. It hurts a little when I pop it back straight, but it's the locking that is what I need to get fixed."

I asked Jimmie about any previous injuries to the left finger, and he said he couldn't think of any. He had been playing the guitar since he was a kid, and he felt like his fingers had really roughened up until the finger started locking up. "Doc, I make a living playing the guitar. I love playing the guitar. This is really freaking me out! What happens if other fingers start locking up? What am I going to do? Go to medical school?"

I asked Jimmie what made his finger lock, and he said, "Just about any time I flex my left middle finger, it locks up. I try to remember to keep it straight, but sometimes when I'm in the moment, I forget and bend it. When I go to straighten it out, it just stays locked up. Most mornings I wake up with that finger in the locked position."

On physical examination, Jimmie was afebrile. His respirations were 18, and his pulse was 64 and regular. His blood pressure was 118/70. Jimmie's head, eyes, ears, nose, throat (HEENT) exam was normal, as was his cardiopulmonary examination. His thyroid was normal, as was his abdominal examination. There was no costovertebral angle (CVA) tenderness. There was no peripheral edema. His low back examination was unremarkable. Visual inspection of the left hand was unremarkable other than some swelling over the flexor tendon of the

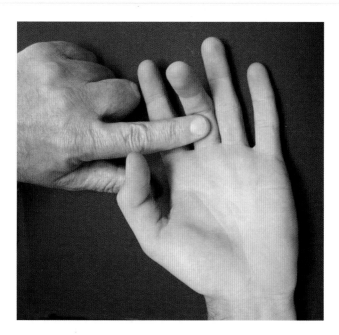

Fig. 13.1   The catching tendon sign for trigger finger. (From Waldman SD. *Physical Diagnosis of Pain: an Atlas of Signs and Symptoms*. Philadelphia: Saunders; 2006:195.)

affected finger, but there was no evidence of infection. The area over the A1 pulley of the left middle finger was tender to palpation. I performed the catching tendon test for trigger finger by having Johnny clench his left hand as tight as he could for 30 seconds and then relax but not open the hand. I then passively extended the affected finger, and I could easily appreciate a locking sensation of the tendon as I slowly tried to actively extend the finger indicating a positive catching tendon sign (Fig. 13.1). With a little increase in pressure to straighten the finger, I felt a pop and the finger straightened.

The right hand examination was normal, as was examination of his other major joints. A careful neurologic examination of the upper and lower extremities revealed there was no evidence of peripheral or entrapment neuropathy, and the deep tendon reflexes were normal. Specifically, there was no evidence of carpal tunnel syndrome, which is common in musicians.

Key Clinical Points—What's Important and What's Not
THE HISTORY

- Triggering of the left middle finger began after overuse from prolonged guitar playing
- Some pain localized to the area of the A1 pulley of the left middle finger

- No other specific traumatic event to the area identified
- No fever or chills
- Finger is in triggered position frequently on waking

THE PHYSICAL EXAMINATION

- Patient is afebrile
- Middle finger of the left hand has a triggering phenomenon
- Swelling and tenderness to palpation of the area over the A1 pulley area
- No evidence of infection
- Catching sensation palpated with extension of the affected finger with sudden pop on forced extension
- Positive catching tendon test on the left middle finger (see Fig. 13.1)

OTHER FINDINGS OF NOTE

- Normal HEENT examination
- Normal cardiovascular examination
- Normal pulmonary examination
- Normal abdominal examination
- No peripheral edema
- Normal upper and lower extremity neurologic examination, motor and sensory examination
- No evidence of carpal tunnel
- Examination of joints other than the left middle finger was normal

 What Tests Would You Like to Order?

The following tests were ordered:
- Plain radiographs of the left hip
- Ultrasound of the left middle finger flexor tendon apparatus

TEST RESULTS

The plain radiographs of the left finger were reported as normal. Ultrasound examination of the left middle finger flexor revealed nodules under the A1 pulley as well as tendinopathy of the flexor tendon as it passed beneath the A1 pulley (Fig. 13.2).

 Clinical Correlation—Putting It All Together

What is the diagnosis?
- Trigger finger

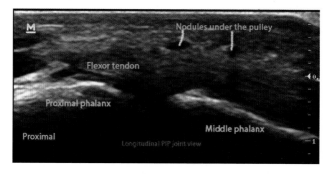

Fig. 13.2   Tigger finger. Longitudinal ultrasound image demonstrating multiple nodules under pulley.

The Science Behind the Diagnosis
ANATOMY

The most common site of pathology in trigger finger is in the flexor tendon and tendon sheath of the flexor digitorum superficialis and profundus muscles of the second to fifth fingers (Fig. 13.3). Sesamoid bones, bone excrescences, and foreign bodies within the tendon sheath at the level of the metacarpal heads may also contribute to the development of trigger finger (Fig. 13.4).

CLINICAL SYNDROME

Trigger finger is caused by inflammation and swelling of the tendon of the flexor digitorum superficialis resulting from compression by the head of the metacarpal bone. Sesamoid bones in this region may also compress and cause trauma to the tendon (Fig. 13.5). Trauma is usually the result of repetitive motion or pressure on the tendon as it passes over these bony prominences. If the inflammation and swelling become chronic, the tendon sheath may thicken, resulting in constriction. Frequently, nodules develop on the tendon, and they can often be palpated when the patient flexes and extends the fingers. Such nodules may catch in the tendon sheath as they pass under a restraining tendon pulley, thus producing a triggering phenomenon that causes the finger to catch or lock (Fig. 13.6). Trigger finger occurs more commonly in females and in patients with diabetes. Patients engaged in repetitive activities such as hammering, gripping a steering wheel, or holding a horse's reins too tightly also have a higher incidence of trigger finger (Fig. 13.7).

SIGNS AND SYMPTOMS

The pain of trigger finger is localized to the distal palm, and tender nodules can often be palpated. The pain is constant and is made worse with active gripping

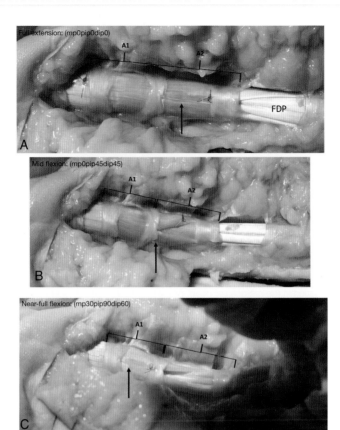

Fig. 13.3 Anatomic dissection of the flexor digitorum superficialis (FDS). (A) Windows have been removed from the distal half of A1 and the proximal A2 preserving a narrow band at the A1/A2 junction. In this posture, marker sutures on FDS overlie locations 1 and 5. An arrow indicates location 4. (B) Tensioning of the FDS has separated the bifurcation with a tendency for the FDS slips to bunch and to rotate around the FDP to a more lateral position. The FDP under tension increases the separation of the FDS slips. The whole tendon mass is thickened in the region of the FDS bifurcation. (C) The thickened FDS bifurcation now lies within the A1 pulley. Further metacarpalphalangeal joint flexion would deliver the thickened tendon mass proximal to A1. Arrow indicates the point on the tendon, which commenced at location 4. (From Chuang XL, Ooi CC, Chin ST, et al. What triggers in trigger finger? The flexor tendons at the flexor digitorum superficialis bifurcation. *J Plast Reconstr Aesth Surg.* 2017;70(10):1411—1419 [Fig. 13.3]. ISSN 1748-6815, https://doi.org/10.1016/j.bjps.2017.05.037.)

motions of the hand. Patients note significant stiffness when flexing the fingers. Sleep disturbance is common, and patients often awaken to find that the finger has become locked in a flexed position (Fig. 13.8).

On physical examination, tenderness and swelling are noted over the tendon, with maximal point tenderness over the head of the metacarpal. Many patients with trigger finger experience a creaking sensation with flexion and extension of the fingers. Range of motion of the fingers may be decreased because of pain, and a triggering phenomenon may be noted. A catching tendon sign may also be

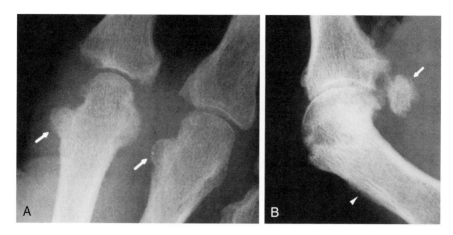

Fig. 13.4 Radiographic abnormalities of the metacarpophalangeal joints. (A) Startling osseous excrescences *(arrows)* around the metacarpal heads are associated with soft tissue swelling, joint space narrowing, and bony erosion and proliferation in the phalanges. (B) At the first metacarpophalangeal joint, irregular bone formation in the metacarpal head, proximal phalanx, and adjacent sesamoid *(arrow)* can be seen. Periostitis of the metacarpal diaphysis is also evident *(arrowhead)*. (From Resnick D. *Diagnosis of Bone and Joint Disorders*. 4th ed. Philadelphia: Saunders; 2000:1087.)

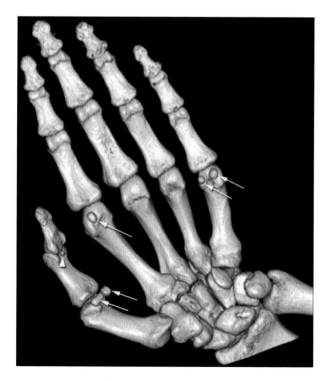

Fig. 13.5 Three-dimensional computed tomography scan demonstrating the sesamoid bones of the hand. (From Ozcanli H, Sekerci R, Keles N. Sesamoid disorders of the hand. *J Hand Surg Am*. 2015;40 (6):1231–2123.)

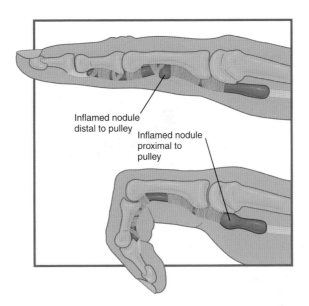

Fig. 13.6 The mechanism of trigger finger. (From Waldman S. *Atlas of Pain Management Injection Techniques*. 4th ed. St. Louis: Elsevier; 2017 [Fig. 82-1].)

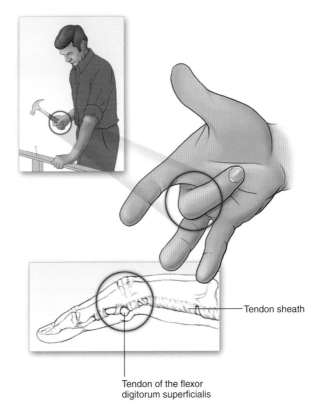

Fig. 13.7 Trigger finger occurs more commonly in females and in patients with diabetes. Patients engaged in repetitive activities such as hammering, gripping a steering wheel, or holding a horse's reins too tightly also have a higher incidence of trigger finger. (From Waldman S. *Atlas of Common Pain Syndromes*. 4th ed. Philadelphia: Elsevier; 2019 [Fig. 56-1].)

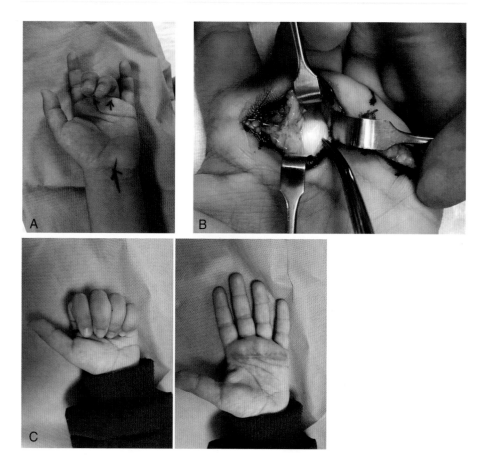

Fig. 13.8   Demonstration of the clinical picture and the operative findings in the left hand. (A) Preoperative appearance of the left hand. Note the locked grade III triggering of the middle and ring fingers. There was also grade II triggering of the index and little fingers. (B) Following the release of pulleys, a large fibrous nodule was seen within the substance of the flexor tendon (at the tip of the mosquito). Note that the senior author uses a single transverse incision across the distal palm to obtain exposure to flexor tendons of adjacent fingers. (C) Postoperative views showing full flexion and extension of the fingers without pain or locking. (From Al-Qattan MM, AlMarshad FA, Ijaz A, et al. Multiple bilateral trigger fingers in a child with neurofibromatosis type I following an acute viral infection: a case report. *Int J Surg Case Rep*. 2020;71:70−72 [Fig. 1].)

elicited by having the patient clench the affected hand for 30 seconds and then relax but not open the hand. If the examiner, after passively extending the affected finger, appreciates a locking, popping, or catching of the tendon as the finger is straightened, the sign is positive (see Fig. 13.1).

TESTING

Plain radiographs are indicated in all patients who present with trigger finger to rule out occult bony disease (Fig. 13.9). Based on the patient's clinical presentation,

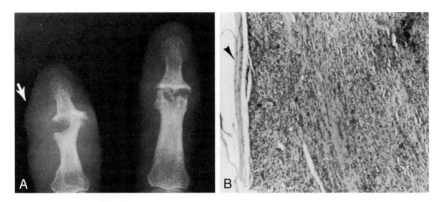

Fig. 13.9   Giant cell tumor of the tendon sheath. (A) In this 56-year-old woman with a 2-year history of pain and gradual swelling of the fingers, a soft tissue mass *(arrow)* can be identified at one distal inter-phalangeal joint. Underlying inflammatory osteoarthritis of the articulations is evident, and this combi-nation of findings would suggest that the mass is a mucous cyst. However, biopsy of the affected joint demonstrated a giant cell tumor of the tendon sheath. (B) Photomicrograph (× 86) in a different patient reveals a tendon capsule tumor *(arrowhead)* associated with moderately vascularized stroma, plump spindle-shaped or ovoid cells, and multinucleated giant cells. (From Resnick D. *Diagnosis of Bone and Joint Disorders*. 4th ed. Philadelphia: Saunders; 2002:4248.)

additional testing may be warranted, including a complete blood count, uric acid level, erythrocyte sedimentation rate, and antinuclear antibody testing. Magnetic resonance imaging (MRI) and ultrasound imaging of the hand are indicated if joint instability or some other abnormality is suspected (Figs. 13.10, 13.11 and 13.12). Color Doppler imaging may aid in the identification of hypervascularity associ-ated with tendinitis (Fig. 13.13).

DIFFERENTIAL DIAGNOSIS

The diagnosis of trigger finger is usually made on clinical grounds. Arthritis or gout of the metacarpal or interphalangeal joints may accompany trigger finger and exacerbate the patient's pain (Fig. 13.14). Occult fractures occasionally con-fuse the clinical presentation.

TREATMENT

Initial treatment of the pain and functional disability associated with trigger fin-ger includes a combination of nonsteroidal antiinflammatory drugs or cyclooxygenase-2 inhibitors and physical therapy. A nighttime splint to protect the fingers may also help relieve the symptoms. If these treatments fail, careful injection of the inflamed flexor apparatus is a reasonable next step. Ultrasound

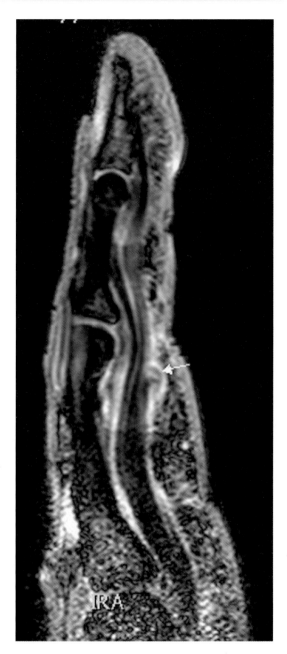

Fig. 13.10 Magnetic resonance T2-weighted sagittal image showing the impinging flexor tendon tag *(arrow)*. (From Couceiro J, Fraga J, Sanmartin M. Trigger finger following partial flexor tendon laceration: magnetic resonance imaging-assisted diagnosis. *Int J Surg Case Rep*. 2015;9:112—114.)

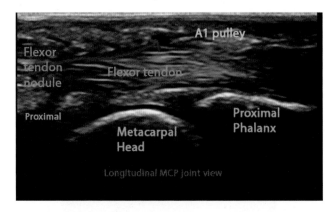

Fig. 13.11   Longitudinal ultrasound image demonstrating a nodule of the flexor tendon in a patient with trigger finger.

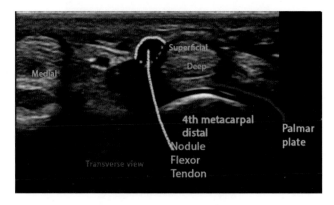

Fig. 13.12   Transverse ultrasound image demonstrating a large nodule of the lateral superficial portion of the flexor tendon in a patient with trigger finger.

guidance may help the operator avoid inadvertent intratendon injection (Figs. 13.15 and 13.16).

Physical modalities, including local heat and gentle range-of-motion exercises, should be introduced several days after the patient undergoes injection. Stretching of the affected tendon and A1 pulley may also be beneficial (Figs. 13.17 and 13.18). Vigorous exercises should be avoided because they will exacerbate the patient's symptoms. Surgical treatment should be considered for patients who fail to respond to the aforementioned treatment modalities.

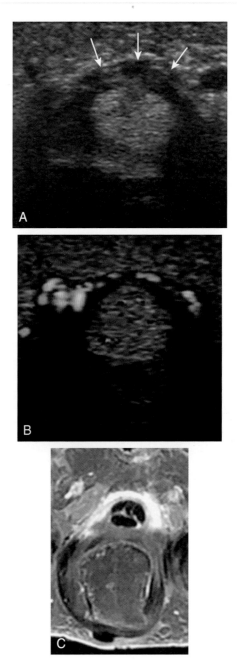

Fig. 13.13   Ultrasound (A) and color Doppler image of trigger finger (B). Arrows indicate hypertrophy of the A1 pulley. Magnetic resonance image with contrast enhancement demonstrates uptake of gadolinium by the inflamed A1 pulley (C). (From Vuillemin V, Guerini H, Bard H, Morvan G: Stenosing tenosynovitis. *J Ultrasound.* 2012;15(1):20–28.)

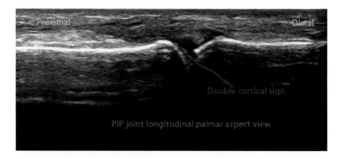

Fig. 13.14 Longitudinal ultrasound image demonstrating the double cortical sign in a patient with poorly controlled gout.

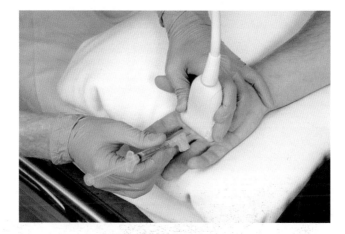

Fig. 13.15 Proper needle placement for ultrasound-guided trigger finger injection.

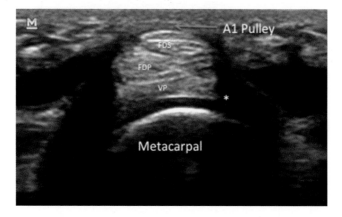

Fig. 13.16 Transverse ultrasound image demonstrating the triangular needle tip target for ultrasound-guided trigger finger injection.

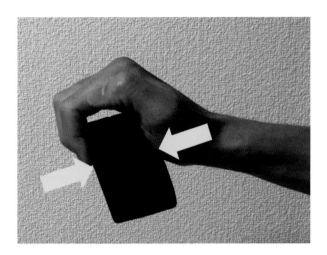

Fig. 13.17 A1 pulley stretching is achieved by fully grasping a block. (From Yamazaki A, Matsuura Y, Kuniyoshi K, et al. A1 pulley stretching treats trigger finger: A1 pulley luminal region under digital flexor tendon traction. *Clin Biomech.* 2020;72:136—140 [Fig. 1]. ISSN 0268-0033, https://doi.org/10.1016/j. clinbiomech.2019.11.018, http://www.sciencedirect.com/science/article/pii/S0268003319300075.)

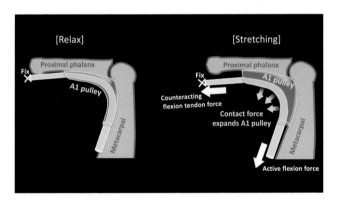

Fig. 13.18 Mechanism of A1 pulley stretching. (From Yamazaki A, Matsuura Y, Kuniyoshi K, et al. A1 pulley stretching treats trigger finger: A1 pulley luminal region under digital flexor tendon traction. *Clin Biomech.* 2020;72:136—140 [Fig. 2]. ISSN 0268-0033, https://doi.org/10.1016/j.clinbiomech.2019.11.018, http://www .sciencedirect.com/science/article/pii/S0268003319300075.)

HIGH-YIELD TAKEAWAYS

- The patient is afebrile, making an acute infectious etiology (e.g., septic arthritis, bursitis, or osteomyelitis) unlikely.
- The patient's symptomatology is the likely result of damage from chronic overuse and irritation of the A1 pulley and associated tendon.

(Continued)

- Since trigger finger is a clinical diagnosis, physical examination and testing should be focused on not only the identification of ligamentous injury, acute arthritis, and tendinitis but also on other pathologic processes that have the potential to harm the patient (e.g., osteomyelitis, osseous tumors, sarcomas).
- The patient has an obvious triggering phenomenon of the finger, which is pathognomonic for the clinical diagnosis of trigger finger.
- Plain radiographs will provide high-yield information and aid in the identification of fractures or other bony abnormalities of the phalanges as well as calcification of the flexor tendons, but ultrasound imaging and MRI will be more useful in identifying soft tissue pathology.
- Dynamic ultrasound imaging may provide identification of the specific anatomic structures responsible for the triggering phenomenon.

Suggested Readings

Akiki RK, Kalliainen LK. Persistent trigger finger due to tendon subluxation. *J Hand Surg.* In press.

Kuczmarski AS, Harris AP, Gil JA, et al. Management of diabetic trigger finger. *J Hand Surg.* 2019;44(2):150–153.

Matzon JL, Lebowitz C, Graham JG, et al. Risk of infection in trigger finger release surgery following corticosteroid injection. *J Hand Surg.* 2020;45(4):310–316.

Quinet MT, Raghavan M, Morris E, et al. Effectiveness of amniotic fluid injection in the treatment of trigger finger: a pilot study. *J Hand Surg (Global Online).* 2020;2(5):301–305.

Waldman SD. Flexor digitorum superficialis and profundus injection for tendinitis and trigger finger. In: *Atlas of Pain Management Injection Techniques.* 4th ed. Philadelphia: Elsevier; 2017:296–300.

Waldman SD. Trigger finger. In: *Waldman's Comprehensive Atlas of Diagnostic Ultrasound of Painful Conditions.* Philadelphia: Wolters Kluwer; 2016:451–456.

Waldman SD. *Trochanteric Bursitis Pain Review.* 2nd ed. Philadelphia: Elsevier; 2017: 303–304.

Waldman SD. Ultrasound-guided injection technique for trigger finger. In: *Waldman's Comprehensive Atlas of Ultrasound Guided Pain Management Injection Techniques.* 2nd ed. Philadelphia: Wolters-Kluwer; 2019:551–558.

Yamazaki A, Matsuura Y, Kuniyoshi K, et al. A1 pulley stretching treats trigger finger: A1 pulley luminal region under digital flexor tendon traction. *Clin Biomech.* 2020;72:136–140.

CHAPTER

14

Chloe Goodheart

A 22-Year-Old Female With Electric Shock–Like Pain and Numbness in the Fingers of the Right Hand

Chloe Goodheart

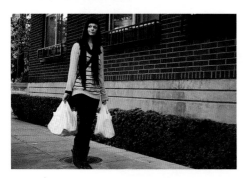

Chloe Goodheart is a 22-year-old hair-stylist with the chief complaint of "I have electric shock—like pain and numbness in my fingers." Chloe stated that over the past several months she began noticing electric shock—like pains, especially in the index and middle fingers on the right. I asked Chloe if she had experienced any numbness or weakness in her hands before, and she replied, "Doc, it's funny that you asked because this happened once before. Not as bad, but similar. Last time it went away after a couple of weeks, but this time, it just won't go away."

I asked Chloe what she thought was causing her symptoms, and she said that it started after she carried home some especially heavy groceries last Thanksgiving. "My parents were coming to visit, and I wanted to fix a really special Thanksgiving meal. I bought this huge frozen turkey and all the trimmings. I guess I bought more food than we needed, but I wanted to make it nice. I had about an 11-block walk from the supermarket, and I have to tell you, those bags got really heavy. I had them double-bag the turkey and the yams and other heavier stuff, but by the time I got home, the handles of the plastic bag had begun to stretch out and cut into my fingers. I got everything home without any bags breaking, but that night my fingers really hurt. The next day, when I was combing out a client's hair, I noticed that I was getting electric shock—like pains that shot into the fingertips of the index and middle fingers of my right hand. I figured it would go away, but if anything, it has gotten worse." I asked Chole what she had tried to make it better, and she said that she used a heating pad at night, and it "seemed to make the shocks a little better. Tylenol PM seemed to help some, at least with sleep." I asked Chloe to describe any numbness she noticed associated with her pain, and she pointed to the distal portion of her right index and middle fingers, especially on the radial side of the fingers. "Doc, the thumb side of my fingers is really numb, and it makes it hard to do the foil when I am coloring a client's hair. It's becoming a real problem." I asked Chloe about any fever, chills, or other constitutional symptoms such as weight loss, night sweats, etc., and she shook her head no. She denied any weakness, but noted that sometimes the electric shocklike pain woke her up at night.

I asked Chloe to point with one finger to show me where it hurt the most. She pointed to the radial aspect of the index and middle fingers and said, "This is where the shocks seem to come from. And I could live with the shocks, but the numbness is really bothering."

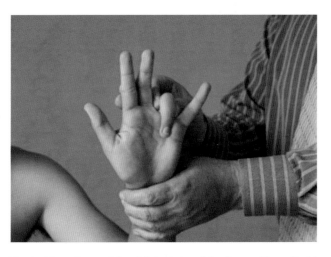

Fig. 14.1   The Allen test for patency of the digital arteries of the fingers. The patient is asked to raise the hand and to tightly flex the affected digit while the examiner occludes the digital arteries on each side of the digit.

On physical examination, Chloe was afebrile. Her respirations were 18, her pulse was 74 and regular, and her blood pressure was 110/68. Chole's head, eyes, ears, nose, throat (HEENT) exam was normal, as was her cardiopulmonary examination. Her thyroid was normal. Her abdominal examination revealed no abnormal mass or organomegaly. There was no costovertebral angle (CVA) tenderness. There was no peripheral edema. Her low back examination was unremarkable. Visual inspection of the right hand was unremarkable. There was no rubor, color, or ecchymosis. There was no obvious infection. The Tinel sign was negative over the right ulnar nerve at the elbow and the right median nerve at the wrist but positive over the digital nerve of the index finger. There was pain on compression of the digital nerves on both the index and middle fingers. The left hand examination was completely normal. Deep tendon reflexes were normal. Chloe's Allen test was negative (Figs. 14.1, 14.2 and 14.3).

Key Clinical Points—What's Important and What's Not

THE HISTORY

- A history of onset of electric shock—like pain and numbness in the right index and middle fingers since carrying heavy plastic bags
- No history of previous significant hand pain
- No fever or chills

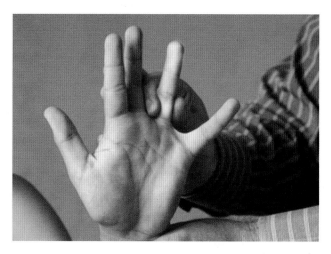

Fig. 14.2   The Allen test for patency of the digital arteries of the fingers. The patient is asked to extend the affected finger; blanching of the finger should be seen, indicating occlusion of digital arteries by the examiner.

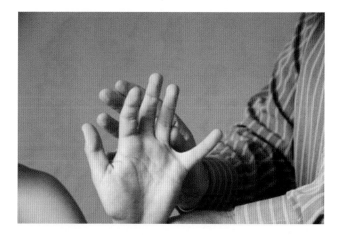

Fig. 14.3   The Allen test for patency of the digital arteries of the fingers. The digital artery on the radial side of the finger is released by the examiner. If the artery is patent, the color will immediately return to the patient's finger. If the color does not return to the finger, the Allen test is considered positive for occlusion of the digital artery on the radial side of the finger.

THE PHYSICAL EXAMINATION

- Patient is afebrile
- Positive Tinel sign at the radial aspect of the index finger
- Tenderness with compression of the digital nerves of the index and middle fingers on the right
- Numbness of the distal index and middle fingers on the right
- No evidence of infection

OTHER FINDINGS OF NOTE

- Negative Tinel sign over ulnar and median nerves at the wrist
- Negative Allen test for patency of the digital arteries of the fingers
- Normal HEENT examination
- Normal cardiovascular examination
- Normal pulmonary examination
- Normal abdominal examination
- No peripheral edema

What Tests Would You Like to Order?

The following tests were ordered:
- Plain radiographs of the hand
- Ultrasound of the right index and middle fingers
- Electromyography (EMG) and nerve conduction velocity testing of the right upper extremity

TEST RESULTS

The plain radiographs of the right hand were reported as normal. Ultrasound examination of the index finger revealed a posttraumatic neuroma of the digital nerve (Fig. 14.4). Segmental nerve conduction testing revealed slowing of the conduction velocity across the lesion.

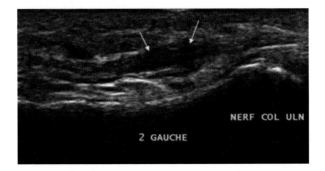

Fig. 14.4 Posttraumatic neuroma of the digital nerve of the index finger. Ultrasound imaging of the index finger, which reveals small swelling on the medial aspect of the index finger due to a posttraumatic neuroma injury, which can be seen on the longitudinal view as a local swelling of the digital nerve *(arrow)*. (From Guerini H, Morvan G, Vuillemin V, et al. Ultrasound of wrist and hand masses. *Diagn Interv Imaging.* 2015;96(12):1247—1260 [Fig. 23]. ISSN 2211-5684, https://doi.org/10.1016/j.diii.2015.10.007, http://www.sciencedirect.com/science/article/pii/S2211568415003630.)

📋 Clinical Correlation—Putting It All Together

What is the diagnosis?

- Plastic bag palsy

The Science Behind the Diagnosis

ANATOMY

The common palmar digital nerves arise from fibers of the median and ulnar nerves (Fig. 14.5). The thumb also has contributions from superficial branches of the radial nerve. The common digital nerves pass along the metacarpal bones and divide as they reach the distal palm. The volar digital nerves supply the majority of sensory innervation to the fingers and run along the ventrolateral

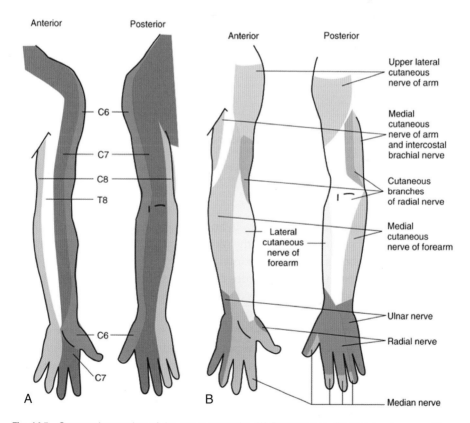

Fig. 14.5 Sensory innervation of the upper extremity. (A) Dermatomes. (B) Peripheral nerves. (From Duffy B, Tubog T. The prevention and recognition of ulnar nerve and brachial plexus injuries. *J PeriAnesth Nurs*. 2017;32(6):636—649 [Fig. 3]. ISSN 1089-9472, https://doi.org/10.1016/j.jopan. 2016.06.005.)

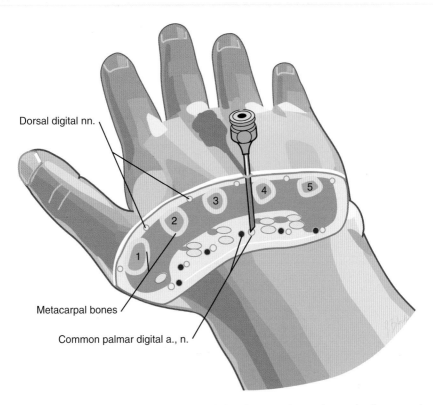

Dorsal digital nn.

Metacarpal bones

Common palmar digital a., n.

Fig. 14.6 The volar digital nerves supply the majority of sensory innervation to the fingers and run along the ventrolateral aspect of the finger beside the digital vein and artery. The smaller dorsal digital nerves contain fibers from the ulnar and radial nerves and supply the dorsum of the fingers as far as the proximal joints. (From Waldman S. *Atlas of Interventional Pain Management*. 5th ed. Philadelphia: Elsevier; 2021 [Fig. 63-3].)

aspect of the finger beside the digital vein and artery (Fig. 14.6). The smaller dorsal digital nerves contain fibers from the ulnar and radial nerves and supply the dorsum of the fingers as far as the proximal joints.

Three common palmar digital arteries find their origin from the convexity of the superficial palmar arch and proceed distally on the second, third, and fourth lumbrical muscles to give off the proper palmar digital arteries, which course along the sides of the index, middle, ring, and little fingers. The proper palmar digital arteries lie just below its corresponding digital nerve, each artery lying just dorsal to its respective digital nerve. The proper palmar digital arteries interconnect and anastamose with the smaller arteries, which supply the interphalangeal joints and pulp of the fingertips (Fig. 14.7). The proper palmar digital arteries also give off dorsal branches, which anastomose with the larger dorsal digital arteries to provide blood supply to the dorsal second and third phalanges as well as the matrix of the respective fingernail matrix. The ulnar side of the little finger is supplied directly from branches of the ulnar artery.

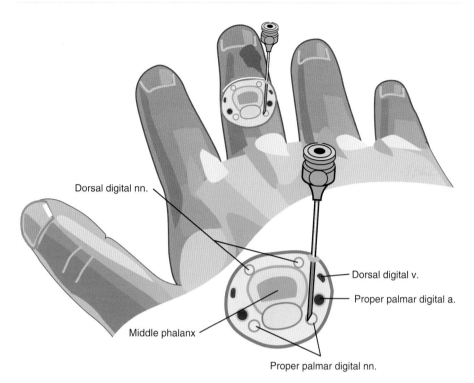

Fig. 14.7 The proper palmar digital arteries interconnect and anastomose with the smaller arteries, which supply the interphalangeal joints and pulp of the fingertips. (From Waldman S. *Atlas of Interventional Pain Management*. 5th ed. Philadelphia: Elsevier; 2021 [Fig. 63-4].)

CLINICAL SYNDROME

Plastic bag palsy is an entrapment neuropathy of the digital nerves caused by compression of the nerves against the bony phalanges by the handles of a plastic bag. The common digital nerves arise from fibers of the median and ulnar nerves. The thumb also has contributions from superficial branches of the radial nerve. The common digital nerves pass along the metacarpal bones and divide as they reach the distal palm. The volar digital nerves supply the majority of sensory innervation to the fingers and run along the ventrolateral aspect of the finger beside the digital vein and artery. The smaller dorsal digital nerves contain fibers from the ulnar and radial nerves and supply the dorsum of the fingers as far as the proximal joints.

Plastic bag palsy has increased in frequency as stores have switched from paper to plastic bags. Compression by the handles of a heavy plastic bag is the inciting cause, and the most common clinical feature is the presence of painful digital nerves at the point of compression (Fig. 14.8). Plastic bag palsy may present in either an acute or a chronic form. Pain may develop from an acute injury to

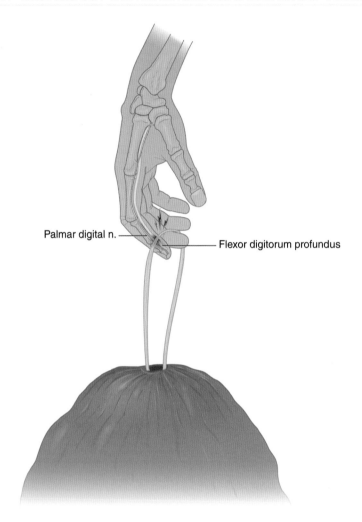

Palmar digital n.

Flexor digitorum profundus

Fig. 14.8   Compression by the handles of a heavy plastic bag is the inciting cause, and the most common clinical feature is the presence of painful digital nerves at the point of compression. (From Waldman S. *Atlas of Pain Management Injection Techniques*. 4th ed. St. Louis: Elsevier; 2017 [Fig. 94-3].)

the nerves after carrying a heavy bag on too few fingers, or it may occur from direct trauma to the soft tissues overlying the digital nerves if the fingers become caught in a bag handle twisted around them. Plastic bag palsy is occasionally seen in homeless people who carry their possessions around in bags and who use the same hand day after day. The affected nerves may be thickened, and inflammation of the nerve and overlying soft tissues may be seen. In addition to pain, patients may complain of paresthesias and numbness just below the point of nerve compromise.

SIGNS AND SYMPTOMS

The pain of plastic bag palsy is constant and is made worse with compression of the affected digital nerves. Patients often note the inability to hold objects with the affected fingers. Sleep disturbance is common.

On physical examination, the patient has tenderness to palpation of the affected digital nerves. Palpation can also cause paresthesias, and continued pressure on the nerves may induce numbness distal to the point of compression. Range of motion of the thumb is normal. With acute trauma to the sesamoid, ecchymosis of the skin overlying the affected digital nerves may be present.

TESTING

Plain radiographs are indicated in all patients who present with plastic bag palsy to rule out occult bony disorders such as bone spurs or cysts that may be compressing the digital nerves (Fig. 14.9). EMG can distinguish other causes of hand numbness. Based on the patient's clinical presentation, additional testing may be indicated, including a complete blood count, uric acid level, erythrocyte sedimentation rate, and antinuclear antibody testing. Magnetic resonance imaging (MRI) and ultrasound imaging of the hand can rule out soft tissue abnormalities, including tumors that may be compressing the digital nerves (Fig. 14.10; see also

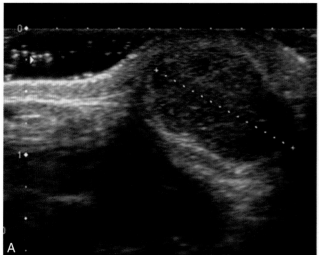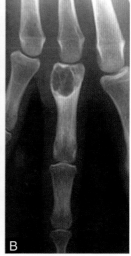

Fig. 14.9 Digital tumor on x-ray and ultrasound (A). Radiographs show bone disease, which was not visible on ultrasound (B). The combination of radiographs with ultrasound is essential in this case. (From Guerini H, Morvan G, Vuillemin V, et al. Ultrasound of wrist and hand masses. *Diagn Interv Imaging*. 2015;96(12):1247—1260 [Fig. 1].)

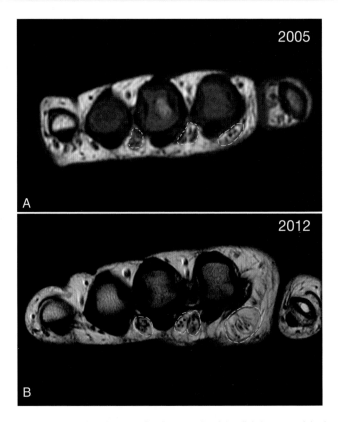

Fig. 14.10   Magnetic resonance imaging revealing lipomatosis of the digital nerves of the hand. Note progression from 2005 (A) to 2012 (B). (From Mahan MA, Niederhauser BD, Amrami KK, et al. Long-term progression of lipomatosis of nerve. *World Neurosurg.* 2014;82(3–4):492–499 [Fig. 2]. ISSN 1878-8750.)

Fig. 14.4). Injection of the digital nerve serves as both a diagnostic and a therapeutic maneuver.

DIFFERENTIAL DIAGNOSIS

The tentative diagnosis of plastic bag palsy is made on clinical grounds and is confirmed by segmental nerve conduction testing. Arthritis, tenosynovitis, or gout of the affected digits may accompany plastic bag palsy and exacerbate the patient's pain. Occult fractures occasionally confuse the clinical presentation, as can tumors of the digital nerves (Figs. 14.11 and 14.12).

TREATMENT

The first step in the treatment of the pain and functional disability associated with plastic bag palsy is to remove the offending compression of the digital nerves.

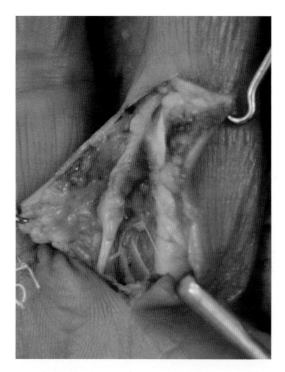

Fig. 14.11   Painful neuroma of the radial digital nerve of the left middle finger. (From Thomsen L, Bellemere P, Loubersac T, et al. Treatment by collagen conduit of painful post-traumatic neuromas of the sensitive digital nerve: a retrospective study of 10 cases. *Chirurgie de la Main*. 2010;29(4):255–262 [Fig. 1].)

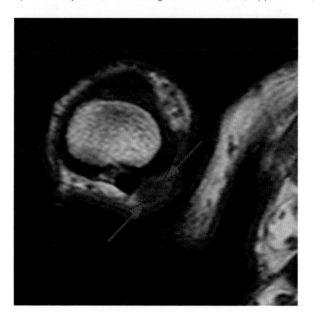

Fig. 14.12   Magnetic resonance imaging demonstrating enlargement of the digital nerve of the thumb consistent with the diagnosis of bowler's thumb, an example of a neuroma of the digital nerve.

Nonsteroidal antiinflammatory drugs, simple analgesics, or cyclooxygenase-2 inhibitors may be prescribed as well. If the patient complains of significant dysesthesias or paresthesias, the addition of gabapentin should be considered. Gabapentin is started at a bedtime dose of 300 mg; it is then titrated upward to 3600 mg in divided doses, as side effects allow. Physical modalities, including local heat and gentle range-of-motion exercises, should be introduced to avoid loss of function. Vigorous exercises should be avoided because they will exacerbate the patient's symptoms. A nighttime splint to protect the fingers may be helpful, and wearing padded gloves can take pressure off the affected digital nerves and overlying soft tissue. If sleep disturbance is present, low-dose tricyclic antidepressants are indicated. If the patient does not respond to these conservative modalities, an ultrasound-guided injection of the affected digital nerve with local anesthetic and steroid is a reasonable next step (Fig. 14.13). Rarely, surgical exploration and neuroplasty of the affected nerves are required for symptomatic relief (Fig. 14.14).

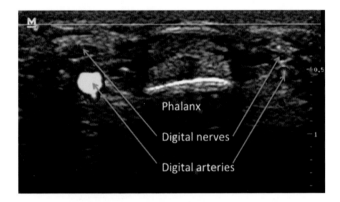

Fig. 14.13   Transverse color Doppler view of the digital artery.

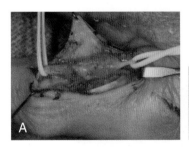
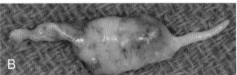

Fig. 14.14   (A) Intraneural ganglion of the dorsal branch of the radial digital nerve of the ring finger. (B) The ganglion was excised with the nerve. (From Naam NH, Carr SB, Massoud AHA. Intraneural ganglions of the hand and wrist. *J Hand Surg.* 2015;40(8):1625–1630.)

HIGH-YIELD TAKEAWAYS

- The patient is afebrile, making an acute infectious etiology unlikely.
- The patient's symptomatology is thought to be the result of prolonged pressure on the right digital nerve.
- Physical examination and testing should be focused on the identification of the various causes of plastic bag palsy.
- The patient exhibits the neurologic and physical examination findings that are highly suggestive of plastic bag palsy.
- The patient's symptoms are unilateral, suggestive of a local process rather than a systemic inflammatory process.
- Plain radiographs will provide high-yield information regarding the bony contents of the joint, but ultrasound imaging and MRI will be more useful in identifying soft tissue pathology that may be responsible for digital nerve compromise.
- EMG and nerve conduction velocity testing will help delineate the location and degree of nerve compromise if digital nerve compromise is suspected.

Suggested Readings

Naam NH, Carr SB, Massoud AHA. Intraneural ganglions of the hand and wrist. *J Hand Surg Am*. 2015;40(8):1625–1630.

Rosenbaum AJ, Leonard G, Mulligan M, et al. Nerve entrapments in musicians. *Nerves Nerve Inj*. 2015;2:665–675.

Waldman SD. Metacarpal and digital nerve block. In: *Atlas of Interventional Pain Management*. 5th ed. Elsevier; 2021:320–324.

Waldman SD. Painful conditions of the wrist and hand. In: *Physical Diagnosis of Pain: An Atlas of Signs and Symptoms*. 3rd ed. Philadelphia: Elsevier; 2016:166.

Waldman SD. Plastic bag palsy. In: *Atlas of Common Pain Syndromes*. 4th ed. Elsevier; 2019:228–230.

Waldman SD. The Wartenberg test for digital nerve entrapment at the elbow. In: *Physical Diagnosis of Pain: An Atlas of Signs and Symptoms*. 4th ed. Philadelphia: Saunders; 2017:133–134.

CHAPTER

15

Vinnie Dang

A 23-Year-Old Bartender With Severe Subungual Pain With Exposure to Cold

LEARNING OBJECTIVES

- Learn the common causes of finger pain.
- Develop an understanding of the anatomy of the digital nerves.
- Develop an understanding of the unique clinical presentation of glomus tumor of the finger.
- Develop an understanding of the differential diagnosis of finger pain.
- Learn how to use physical examination to identify glomus tumor of the hand.
- Develop an understanding of the treatment options for glomus tumor.

Vinnie Dang

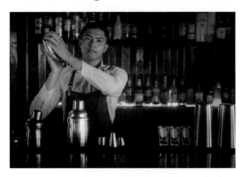

Vinnie Dang is a 23-year-old bartender with the chief complaint of "every time my index finger gets cold, I feel like somebody is stabbing it with a knife." Vinnie stated that for the last couple of months, any time his right index finger gets cold, he gets a sharp, stabbing pain underneath his finger-nail. "Doctor, I dread it when someone pulls the 007, as I know it's going to hurt." I asked, "What's a 007?" Vinnie grinned and said, "You know, Doctor, 'shaken not stirred.'" I must have had a blank look on my face because Vinnie laughed and said, "Doctor, when you make a martini, you put the ingredients into a cocktail shaker and you have to hold the top and bottom together with your hand as you shake it. The idea is to get the liquor super cold. Once you get it shaken, you strain out the ice as you pour it into the martini glass. Not much of a drinker, are you, Doc?" I laughed and said, "Not really, but I got the general idea." Vinnie said, "Doctor, I consider myself a pretty tough guy. You know I was in the army right out of high school. But any time my index finger gets cold, the pain is so bad I want to cry. It really, really hurts!"

I asked Vinnie if he had experienced any pain, numbness, or weakness in either hand before this started, and he shook his head and replied, "Doc, the pain is right under my fingernail. I can see a little blue spot under the nail. And lately, the nail has gotten kind of gnarly looking. I don't remember injuring the nail, but I guess I could have done it in my sleep." I asked, "How is your sleep?" Vinnie said, "It's fine. The nail is sensitive to touch, but unless I roll over on my finger, it is fine." I asked what made the pain better, and he said, "Keeping the finger away from anything cold."

I asked Vinnie to show me where the pain was, and he pointed to the nail of his right index finger. I could immediately see the nail deformity. I asked Vinnie about any fever, chills, or other constitutional symptoms such as weight loss, night sweats, etc., and he shook his head no. He also denied any other musculo-skeletal or systemic symptoms.

On physical examination, Vinnie was afebrile. His respirations were 18, his pulse was 74 and regular, and his blood pressure was 124/76. Vinnie's head, eyes, ears, nose, throat (HEENT) exam was normal, as was his thyroid exam. Auscultation of his carotids revealed no bruits, and the pulses in all four extremi-ties were normal. He had a regular rhythm without abnormal beats. His cardiac exam was otherwise unremarkable. His abdominal examination revealed no abnormal mass or organomegaly. There was no peripheral edema. His low back

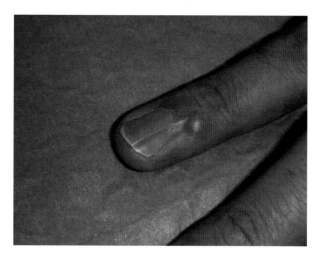

Fig. 15.1 Glomus tumor of index finger. (From Smilevitch DF, Chaput B, Grolleau J-L, et al. Improvement in quality of life after surgery for glomus tumors of the fingers. *Chirurgie de la Main.* 2014;33(5):330—335 [Fig. 1B]. ISSN 1297-3203, https://doi.org/10.1016/j.main.2014.07.001, http://www.sciencedirect.com/science/article/pii/S1297320314001012.)

examination was unremarkable, although flexion of the lumbar spine caused some pain in the right buttocks. There was no costovertebral angle (CVA) tenderness. Visual inspection of the nail of the right index finger revealed a small bluish discolored area and deformity of the nail (Fig. 15.1). There was no rubor or color and no evidence of ecchymosis or obvious fungal infection of the nail. Pressure on the nail caused Vinnie to say, "You're right on it, Doc! That's it." I performed an ice water test, which took a fair amount of convincing, and it was positive within about 15 seconds (Fig. 15.2). Vinnie said, "No more of that, Doc. How about I mash your index finger with a ballpeen hammer? Because that's how much it hurts."

A careful neurologic examination of both the upper and lower extremities was normal. Deep tendon reflexes were physiologic throughout. "Sorry, Vinnie, I am pretty sure I know what is causing the pain, and it is pretty straightforward to fix."

Key Clinical Points—What's Important and What's Not

THE HISTORY

- History of lancinating subungual pain with exposure to cold
- Pain made worse with pressure on the affected nail
- Discoloration under the nail
- Nail deformity noted

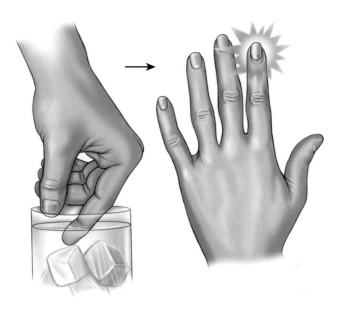

Fig. 15.2 Glomus tumor is characterized by (1) excruciating distal digit pain, (2) ability to trigger the pain by palpation, and (3) marked intolerance to cold. It is easily diagonsed by the ice water test. (From Waldman SD. *Atlas of Uncommon Pain Syndromes*. Philadelphia: Saunders; 2003:108.)

- No symptoms in the left upper extremity
- No fever or chills
- No history of recent trauma

THE PHYSICAL EXAMINATION

- Patient is afebrile
- Subungual discoloration of the right index finger
- Nail deformity of the right index finger (see Fig. 15.1)
- Pain reproduced with pressure on the affected nail (Love test)
- Positive ice water test (see Fig. 15.2)

OTHER FINDINGS OF NOTE

- Normal HEENT examination
- Normal cardiovascular examination
- Normal pulmonary examination
- Normal abdominal examination
- No peripheral edema

What Tests Would You Like to Order?

The following tests were ordered:
- X-ray of the right hand
- Ultrasound of the right index finger
- Magnetic resonance imaging (MRI) of the index finger

TEST RESULTS

X-ray of the right hand revealed bony erosion of the distal phalanx from a paraungual glomus tumor (Fig. 15.3). Ultrasound and color Doppler examination of the distal phalanx revealed a hypoechoic nodule causing bony scalloping on the phalanx (Fig. 15.4). MRI of the index finger revealed a glomus tumor (Fig. 15.5).

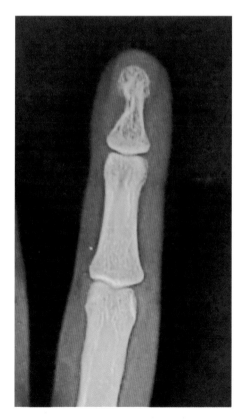

Fig. 15.3 Plain radiograph showing bony erosion on distal phalanx because of the paraungual glomus tumor in 25-year-old female. (From Morey VM, Garg B, Kotwal PP. Glomus tumours of the hand: review of literature. *J Clin Orthop Trauma*. 2016;7(4):286–291 [Fig. 2]. ISSN 0976-5662, https://doi.org/10.1016/j.jcot.2016.04.006, http://www.sciencedirect.com/science/article/pii/S0976566216300339.)

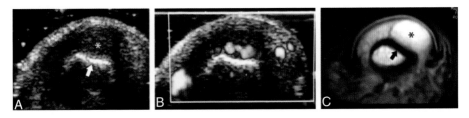

Fig. 15.4 Subungual glomus tumor. (A) B mode ultrasound shows hypoechoic nodule *(*)* causing bony scalloping on the phalanx *(arrow)*. (B) On Doppler mode ultrasound, the mass displays incomplete hypervascularization but wider vascular areas different from the vessels of the naturally hypervascularized nail bed. (C) T1-weighted magnetic resonance image obtained after intravenous administration of a gadolinium chelate shows bony scalloping *(arrow)*. The glomus tumor *(*)* shows marked enhancement. (From Guerini H, Morvan G, Vuillemin V, et al. Ultrasound of wrist and hand masses. *Diagn Interv Imaging*. 2015;96(12):1247−1260 [Fig. 10]. ISSN 2211-5684, https://doi.org/10.1016/j.diii. 2015.10.007, http://www.sciencedirect.com/science/article/pii/S2211568415003630.)

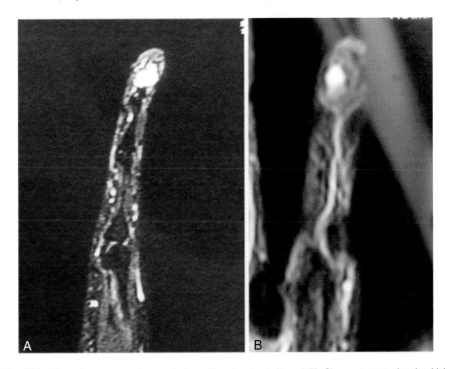

Fig. 15.5 Magnetic resonance images in two different patients (A and B). Glomus tumors showing high signal intensity on T2-weighted images. (From Morey VM, Garg B, Kotwal PP. Glomus tumours of the hand: review of literature. *J Clin Orthop Trauma*. 2016;7(4):286−291 [Fig. 3]. ISSN 0976-5662, https://doi. org/10.1016/j.jcot.2016.04.006, http://www.sciencedirect.com/science/article/pii/S0976566216300339.)

📋 Clinical Correlation—Putting It All Together

What is the diagnosis?
- Glomus tumor

The Science Behind the Diagnosis

ANATOMY

The glomus tumor is a tumor of the glomus body. It is comprised of the collecting venule, anastomotic vessel, and afferent arteriole. Although glomus tumors can occur anywhere in the body, they occur most commonly under the fingernails. The vast majority of glomus tumors are benign, but malignant degeneration is not unheard of (Fig. 15.6).

CLINICAL SYNDROME

Glomus tumor of the hand is an uncommon cause of distal finger pain. It is the result of tumor formation of the glomus body, which is a neuromyoarterial apparatus whose function is to regulate peripheral blood flow in the digits. Most patients with glomus tumor are women, 30 to 50 years of age. The pain is severe in intensity, lancinating, and boring. The tumor frequently involves the nail bed and may invade the distal phalanx. Patients with glomus tumor of the hand exhibit the classic triad of excruciating distal finger pain, cold intolerance, and tenderness to palpation of the affected digit. Multiple glomus tumors are present in approximately 25% of patients diagnosed with this disease. Glomus tumors also can occur in the foot and occasionally in other parts of the body. They are usually benign, but malignant degeneration can occur.

SIGNS AND SYMPTOMS

The diagnosis of glomus tumor of the hand is based primarily on three points in the patient's clinical history: (1) excruciating pain localized to a distal digit, (2) the ability

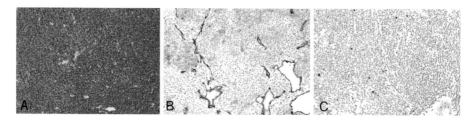

Fig. 15.6 Histology of a glomus tumor with intermediate malignant potential. On hematoxylin-eosin stain (A and B), the tumor was well limited by a thin fibrous capsule, and assumed a vaguely nodular and angiocentric architecture, interspersed with congestive capillaries of various size, admixed with a few smooth muscle bundles. A reticulin stain highlighted a delicate weaving surrounding every tumor cell individually (C). Immunohistochemistry showed a strong and diffuse positivity to smooth muscle actin, accompanied by a weaker staining to CD34 in 30% of the tumor cells. MIB-1 proliferation index was close to 1%. (From Drabent P, Bielle F, Bernat I, et al. Epineural glomus tumor of the posterior interosseous nerve: case report. *J Clin Neurosci.* 2020;74:232–234 [Fig. 2D-F]. ISSN 0967-5868, https://doi .org/10.1016/j.jocn.2019.12.062, http://www.sciencedirect.com/science/article/pii/S0967586819321526.)

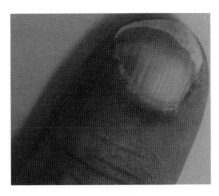

Fig. 15.7   The classic bluish discoloration of the nail plate is seen on the right proximal corner of the nail in a patient with a subungual glomus tumor. (From McDermott EM, Weiss AP. Glomus tumors. *J Hand Surg Am*. 2006;31:1397–1400.)

to trigger the pain by palpating the area (Love test), and (3) marked intolerance to cold. The pain of glomus tumor can be reproduced by placing the affected digit in a glass of ice water (see Fig. 15.2). If glomus tumor is present, the characteristic lancinating, boring pain occurs within 30 to 60 seconds. Placing other unaffected fingers of the same hand in ice water does not trigger the pain in the affected finger. Hildreth test also is useful in the diagnosis of glomus tumor. It is performed by placing a tourniquet proximal to the area of suspected tumor. As the distal area becomes ischemic, the sharp lancinating pain characteristic of glomus tumor will occur. Nail bed ridging is present in many patients with glomus tumor of the hand, and a small blue or dark red spot at the base of the nail is visible in 10% to 15% of patients with the disease (Figs. 15.7 and 15.8; see also Fig. 15.1). The patient with glomus tumor of the hand frequently wears a finger protector on the affected digit and guards against hitting the digit on anything to avoid triggering the pain.

TESTING

MRI of the affected digit often reveals the actual glomus tumor and may reveal erosion or a perforating lesion of the phalanx beneath the tumor (Fig. 15.9). The tumor appears as a very high and homogeneous signal on T2-weighted images. The bony changes associated with glomus tumor of the hand also may appear on plain radiographs if a careful comparison of the corresponding contralateral digit is made. Radionuclide bone scan also may reveal localized bony destruction. The ice water test mentioned earlier helps the clinician strengthen the diagnosis. Based on the patient's clinical presentation, additional tests, including complete blood cell count, uric acid level, erythrocyte sedimentation rate, and antinuclear antibody testing, may be indicated. Electromyography is indicated if coexistent ulnar or carpal tunnel syndrome is suspected. Surgical exploration of the affected digit and nail bed often is necessary to confirm the diagnosis (Fig. 15.10).

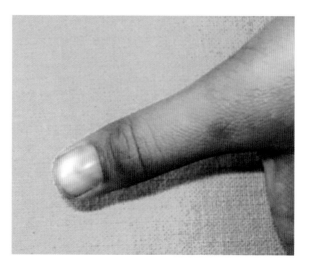

Fig. 15.8   Bluish pink discoloration of the nail plate of left thumb because of a subungual glomus tumour in a 21-year-old female. (From Morey VM, Garg B, Kotwal PP. Glomus tumours of the hand: review of literature. *J Clin Orthop Trauma*. 2016;7(4):286–291 [Fig. 1]. ISSN 0976-5662, https://doi.org/10.1016/j.jcot.2016.04.006, http://www.sciencedirect.com/science/article/pii/S0976566216300339.)

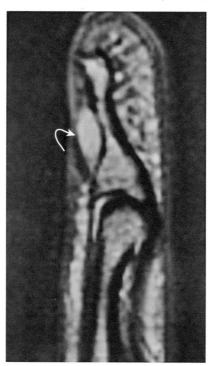

Fig. 15.9   Glomus tumor. Fast T2 sagittal image, finger. There is a small, high signal mass *(curved arrow)* on the dorsum of the distal phalanx, causing bone erosion. (From Kaplan PA, Helms CA, Dussault R, et al. *Musculoskeletal MRI*. Philadelphia: Saunders, 2001:273.)

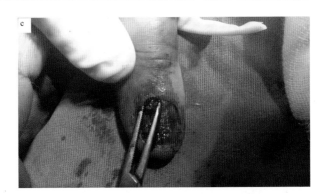

Fig. 15.10 Dissection and excision of capsulated glomus tumor after nail removal. (From ElSherif M, Abonnour M. Outcome of transungual surgical approach with synthetic nail shield in the treatment of digital glomus tumors: a retrospective study. *JPRAS Open.* 2020 [Fig. 1C]. ISSN 2352-5878, https://doi.org/10.1016/j.jpra.2020.09.004, http://www.sciencedirect.com/science/article/pii/S2352587820300395.)

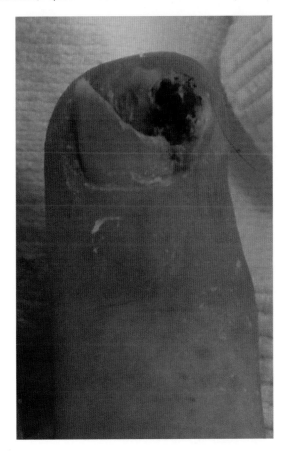

Fig. 15.11 Subungual malignant melanoma. (From Hinchcliff KM, Pereira C. Subungual tumors: an algorithmic approach. *J Hand Surg.* 2019;44(7):588—598 [Fig. 12]. ISSN 0363-5023, https://doi.org/10.1016/j.jhsa.2018.12.015, http://www.sciencedirect.com/science/article/pii/S0363502318304350.)

DIFFERENTIAL DIAGNOSIS

The triad of localized excruciating distal digit pain, tenderness to palpation, and cold intolerance makes the diagnosis apparent to an astute clinician. Glomus tumor of the hand must be distinguished from other causes of localized hand pain, including subungual melanoma and osteoid osteoma. If a history of trauma is present, fracture, osteomyelitis, tenosynovitis, and foreign body synovitis should be considered. If there is no history of trauma, then gout, other crystal monarthropathies, tumors, and diseases of the nail and nail bed should be considered. Reflex sympathetic dystrophy should be distinguishable from glomus tumor of the hand because the pain of reflex sympathetic dystrophy is less

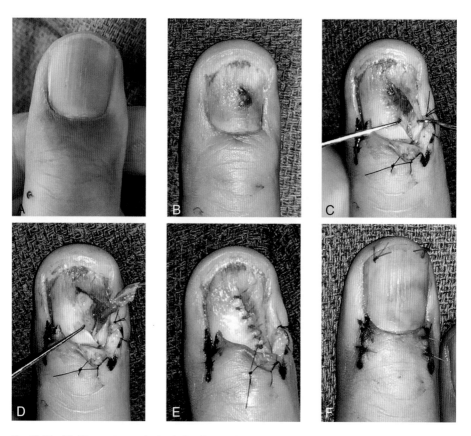

Fig. 15.12 (A) Glomus tumor in the index finger of a woman, presenting with a small bluish, painful lesion. (B–D) Excision of the tumor through a nail plate removal approach. (E) Primary closure of the sterile matrix with absorbable suture to prevent future nail deformity. (F) Stenting of the eponychial fold with the removed nail plate to prevent scarring and improve the chances for normal nail regrowth. (From Hinchcliff KM, Pereira C. Subungual tumors: an algorithmic approach. *J Hand Surg*. 2019;44(7): 588–598 [Fig. 5].)

localized and is associated with trophic skin and nail changes and vasomotor and sudomotor abnormalities. Raynaud syndrome usually involves the entire hand, and the ice water test mentioned typically triggers pain if the "unaffected" finger is tested. Other painful subungual tumors include eccrine spiradenoma, leiomyoma, squamous cell carcinomas, angioleiomyoma, hemangioma, and neuromas. Although not usually painful, subungual malignant melanoma should always be included in the differential diagnosis because if its poor prognosis (Fig. 15.11).

TREATMENT

The mainstay of treatment of glomus tumor is surgical removal (Fig. 15.12). Medication management is uniformly disappointing. Injection of the affected digit in the point of maximal tenderness may provide temporary relief of the pain of glomus tumor and block the positive ice water test response, further strengthening the diagnosis.

HIGH-YIELD TAKEAWAYS

- The patient is afebrile, making an acute infectious etiology unlikely.
- The patient's symptomatology is consistent with the classic clinical presentation of subungual glomus tumor.
- Physical examination and testing should be focused on the identification of other pathologic processes that may mimic the clinical diagnosis of subungual glomus tumor, in particular malignant melanoma.
- The ice water test is highly specific for the diagnosis of glomus tumor.
- X-ray, ultrasound, and MRI of the affected digit may confirm the diagnosis or identify unexpected causes of the patient's pain symptomatology.

Suggested Readings

Constantinesco A, Arbogast S, Foucher G, et al. Detection of glomus tumor of the finger by dedicated MRI at 0.1 T. *Magn Reson Imaging*. 1994;12:1131–1134.

Dilger AE, Cramer J, Dutra J. Thyroid mass from a malignant glomus tumor: case report and literature review. *Otolaryngol Case Rep*. 2017;5:28–30.

Drabent P, Bielle F, Bernat I, et al. Epineural glomus tumor of the posterior interosseous nerve: case report. *J Clin Neurosci*. 2020;74:232–234.

Gandon F, Legaillard Ph, Brueton R, et al. Forty-eight glomus tumours of the hand: retrospective study and four-year follow-up. *Ann Chir Main Memb Super*. 1992;11:401–405.

Gombos Z, Fogt F, Zhang PJ. Intraosseous glomus tumor of the great toe: a case report with review of the literature. *J Foot Ankle Surg*. 2008;47:299–301.

Hinchcliff KM, Pereira C. Subungual tumors: an algorithmic approach. *J Hand Surg*. 2019;44(7):588–598.

Jaoude JFA, Farah AR, Sargi Z, et al. Glomus tumors: report on eleven cases and a review of the literature. *Chirurg Main*. 2000;19:243–252.

McDermott EM, Weiss C. Glomus tumors. *J Hand Surg Am*. 2006;31:1397–1400.

Waldman SD. Glomus tumor of the finger. In: *Atlas of Uncommon Pain Syndromes*. 4th ed. Philadelphia: Elsevier; 2020:179–181.

Page numbers followed by '*f*' indicate figures, '*t*' indicate tables and '*b*' indicate boxes.

A

Abductor pollicis longus tendon, 64,
    79–80
  angle of incidence, 67*f*
  de Quervain tenosynotis, 67*f*
Adductor pollicis brevis, 42
Allen test, 204*f*, 205*f*
Arthritis
  carpal joints, 7*f*
  Watson stress test for, 106*f*
  wrist, 8–10
Avascular necrosis (AVN), scaphoid
    bone, 150, 150*f*
  anatomic snuff box, 153*f*
  differential diagnosis, 154, 156*b*
  posteroanterior radiograph, 154*f*
  predisposing factors, 152*b*
  signs and symptoms, 152–153
  treatment, 154–157

B

Bugaboo wrist. *See* Intersection
    syndrome

C

Calcification
  anteroposterior and oblique
    radiographs, 168*f*

Calcification (*Continued*)
  pisiform, 161–162, 161*f*, 165*f*
Calcific tendinitis, flexor carpi ulnaris,
    161–162, 161*f*
Carpal boss
  differential diagnosis, 140–143,
    141*f*, 142*f*, 143*b*
  dorsal ganglion, 134*f*
  hunchback sign, 135*f*, 136
  inflamed bursa, 143*f*
  injection technique for, 144*f*
  radiographic manifestations,
    138*f*
  signs and symptoms, 138–139
  treatment, 144
  with wrist flexion, 139*f*
Carpal joints arthritis, 7*f*
Carpal tunnel anatomy, 31*f*
Carpal tunnel syndrome, 101–102
  anatomy, 28–29, 32*f*
  conditions associated with, 34*b*
  cyst, 35*f*
  diagnosis, 28
  electromyography, 35
  magnetic resonance imaging axial
    section, 29*f*
  opponens weakness test for,
    25*f*
  Phalen maneuver, 34–35
  positioning of hand and wrist
    during keyboarding, 33*f*

E